THE BUSY PARENT'S GUIDE TO RAISING SUPER HEALTHY KIDS

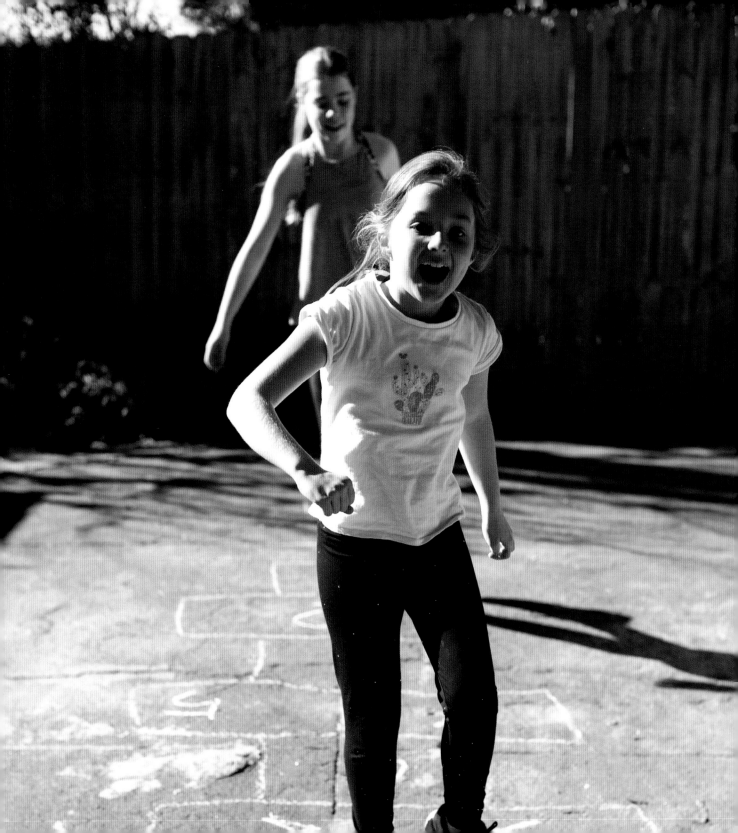

THE BUSY PARENT'S GUIDE TO RAISING SUPER HEALTHY KIDS

Nicole Monteforte and Shane Byrne

NEW
HOLLAND

Contents

PART FOUR: DON'T STRESS OUT!

PART FIVE: LET'S JOIN THE DOTS

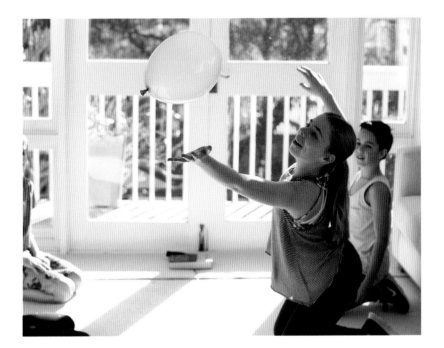

DEDICATION

This book is dedicated to our families, children and good friends, who have given us the support, unconditional love and courage to write this book and share our beliefs with the world.

FOREWORD

by Professor Kerryn Phelps AM MBBS (Syd), FRACGP

Obesity is considered to be at epidemic levels and many children with suboptimal nutrition and an unhealthy lifestyle face a future of preventable chronic disease.

I have known Nic Monteforte personally and through the fitness industry for nearly 20 years. In that time Nic has worked closely with Shane Byrne with a shared passion to contribute to the fitness and wellbeing industry.

When it comes to the health and wellbeing of children, both Nic and Shane are parents who believe in living their philosophy. They make sure their own children are physically active and eat well.

Parents leading busy lives can run out of puff when it comes to new ideas for keeping their children physically active, and some fresh ideas from two experienced fitness professionals are very welcome.

My daughter, Jaime Rose Chambers, an experienced dietitian, has contributed her nutritional expertise to this book. Jaime works with children and parents to help them change their children's unhealthy eating habits, sometimes passed down through generations. Our first lessons about what foods to buy and to prepare come from our childhood homes. It is no secret where Jaime got her early awareness of the link between practical nutrition and health! Let's face it: parents are in control of what food is in the house, what is prepared for meals and what goes into their children's school lunch boxes.

There is no more important responsibility for a parent than to provide their children with the ingredients for a healthy and happy life.

In a world where children are spending more and more time sitting in front of a computer screen, playing with their iPads or texting on their phones, it is more important than ever to ensure that good eating habits and regular exercise are integral parts of your children's lives.

The Busy Parent's Guide to Raising Super-Healthy Kids is a wonderful resource for parents looking for new inspiration.

WHO ARE WE?

NIC MONTEFORTE, Bachelor of Physical Education

Nicole Monteforte is an exceptionally motivated, positive and engaging person, and is a mother of two healthy and active teenagers. Nic successfully ran a multi-million-dollar fitness company, during which time she led many corporate teams to immense success. Her experiences provided an unrivaled insight into human behavior, which has enabled Nic to effectively apply and adapt key business leadership principles to child rearing. This along with her experience and passion in the health space, has seen her expand into becoming focused on a holistic approach which now also includes food and nutrition. The impact of the obesity epidemic on kids and their families, coupled with the realization that parents are feeling powerless to help their children, was the catalyst behind Nic deciding to write this no-holds-barred guide for parents and carers.

SHANE BYRNE, Bachelor of Human Movement

Shane Byrne has an intricate knowledge of the human body, having worked in the fitness industry for more than 20 years. His unique approach to wellness saw him evolve from a personal trainer with a prestigious client base, to a key executive in a multi-million-dollar national fitness chain. Shane's realistic attitude and appreciation of the pressures that parents face each and every day (something he learned first-hand as a father of two), was the motivation for him to explore ways to create positive change. Shane believes there is no need for our kids to be overweight. He is passionate about teaching both parents and kids how easy it is to become healthy and stay that way for life.

JAIME ROSE CHAMBERS, Accredited Practising Dietitian and Nutritionist

Jaime has spent her career working in private practice. She is also the nutrition leader for the Go4Fun, which is a successful publicly funded nutrition, exercise and healthy lifestyle program for children. Over the past seven years, Jaime has delivered 18 programs, which has helped around 200 kids and their families successfully change their home environment, enhance their nutrition, improve their eating habits and get them more active. Jaime has a passion for food, cooking, and educating others about the powerful affect that eating can have on the human body and how this can be manipulated for positive and permanent change.

A WORD FROM OUR EXERCISE SPECIALISTS, NIC MONTEFORTE AND SHANE BYRNE

The world we live in is busy. Global obesity and the health issues that result are a very sad reality. In fact, based on present trends we can predict that by the time they reach the age of 20, our kids will have a shorter life expectancy than earlier generations – largely due to the impact of obesity.

Obesity, is defined by the World Health Organization as an abnormal or excessive amount of fat accumulation that can have a negative impact on a person's health. It typically is identified using BMI or body mass index as a rough guide, which is a simple calculation of a persons weight in kilograms divided by their height squared in meters or kg/m2. It is important for the child's BMI to be compared to the percentile charts for other children of their age and gender.

But, as parents, this is a trend that we can control within our own family.

The goal of this book is to provide super-busy parents with some much-needed support, through the provision of some simple, practical and effective strategies. This book aims to help you see how achievable good health really is, even when you think you simply don't know how to fit it in. Before we get into the nitty gritty, here are a few startling facts:

- Between 10–15 per cent of the world's childhood population (defined as 5–17yrs) are obese. This equates to 43 million children worldwide who are classed as obese (BMI greater than 30 per cent).
- In 1990, this percentage was 4.2 per cent. Meaning that the childhood obesity rate has increased by more than 300 per cent in the last 25 years.
- If these levels continue, by 2025 in the developed countries, close to 80 per cent of all adults and one third of all children will be overweight or obese.
- Obesity has overtaken smoking as the leading cause of premature death and illness in the Western world. Obesity has become the single biggest threat to public health globally.
- The average child in the developed countries spends 50 per cent of their free time watching television.
- Children who have TV sets in their bedrooms are also more likely to gain excess weight than children who don't.
- The obesity epidemic now costs the world $2 TRILLION a year!!

The truth is, we are all in this together. But together, we can all make a difference and arrest these alarming health trends along with our peace of mind.

PART ONE

You Are Not Alone

CHAPTER
ONE

Big Kids In The Park

"You Are Not Alone"

Are you one of the many parents who feel worried about their child being one of the larger kids on the swings at the local park?

When sitting at school assembly, do you feel concerned because your child is one of the biggest kids in the class?

When you ask your children what's wrong, do they say they're being picked on by other kids, for being fat? Are they being isolated because they don't get involved in school sports or because they find it hard to keep up in the playground?

Or maybe you've noticed your child has become more quiet and introverted? Do you feel like you are having fewer conversations with your kids, or perhaps you feel like they've lost the bright spark they used to have?

Do you wish you could talk to other parents and say "I don't know what to do?" or "I feel like I've tried everything" or even, "please don't judge, it's not their fault"?

If any of these scenarios ring true, then you're probably also feeling confused and unsure about how to begin to improve the situation and help your child.

The brutal truth is; parenting can feel overwhelming. And it's no wonder. We live in a time-poor society where fast food is easier and sometimes cheaper than cooking from scratch; nutritional advice is available in abundance but is often conflicting and confusing; we feel stressed and under pressure – it's no surprise our health and the health of our family can take a back seat in preference to just getting through each day.

If you are feeling powerless and confused about how to help the most precious people in your world, then rest assured you're not alone. When it comes to kids' health, parents are reading everything they can find in a bid to help them do things differently. Some advice says "don't give your kids soft drinks because they are full of sugar", so you give them diet soft drinks instead. Then you find out that diet soft drinks don't contain real sugar but are full of other dangerous chemicals that prevent your child from losing weight. So, you quit the diet soft drinks and give them fruit juice instead. But then the next article you read explains how bottled fruit juice has just as much sugar as soft drinks, and even though they may be natural sugars they can still have a detrimental health impact on your kids. No wonder you feel more confused than ever!

The next logical step is to start teaching your kids coping strategies to deal with bullies, in anticipation of them having to constantly deal with rejection and being singled out.

It's even possible that you, yourself, may also be gaining weight. You may even be fighting with your partner a lot more who – along with you – is feeling exhausted and run down from all the stress and anxiety.

Well, despair no longer! Because this book holds the solutions to help you regain your power and put an end to all of those worries.

If you would like to have a healthy and active family who has the energy to do all the things they want to, and the enthusiasm to set and achieve goals throughout life, then keep reading.

If you would you like to understand how to help your kids (and the rest of the family – including yourself) flourish and thrive, to become healthy, happy and successful, then this book is for you.

The reality is, living healthier and happier doesn't have to be a difficult or complicated process; and it certainly need not be confusing. This book has been specifically designed to provide you with practical solutions to help you shed the confusion and regain your power and health, and the health and happiness of your family.

By sharing with you all the secrets we hold, we can help your kids (and you) drop the excess kilos and become healthier and happier for life!

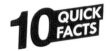

Here are 10 lesser-known facts about health and wellness. And these are just the beginning – there are plenty more of these golden nuggets of information, which you'll learn as you progress through this book.

1. We are born with a certain number of fat cells and when we gain weight, those fat cells fill with fat. When they are so full they can't get any bigger, our body makes more fat cells. The problem is, when we lose weight, we now have more fat cells and so are more prone to weight gain. This can make maintaining a healthy weight a little more challenging.

2. When we say "you're not alone", we mean it! Currently 15 per cent of children across the globe are obese.

3. Being overweight is not just about aesthetics; it can be dangerous because it is linked to a wide range of health issues.

4. Alarmingly, across the globe, in excess of 50 per cent of obese adolescents grow up to become obese adults.

5. The rate of obesity significantly increases in children who watch more than two hours of 'screen time' per day (the definition of 'screen time' includes TV, computer and video games).

6. Overweight children are at a much greater risk of being bullied at school than children of a healthy weight.

7. Being physically active does not rely on your financial status. Whether you are wealthy or struggling to pay bills, your children can be fit and healthy. It doesn't cost money to get your children moving around on a regular basis.

8. It only takes 21 days to form a habit, which is not a lot of time in relation to one's lifetime!

9. Sugar and sugar derivatives can be enormous barriers to weight loss.

10. By the end of this book, you will have learned how to have a healthy and happy family!

So how are you feeling now? Hopefully, a little more hopeful because you understand that you are not alone in your confusion, and that you are about to discover the secrets that will successfully help you say "goodbye" to the helplessness, and "hello" to some permanent and positive changes.

Let's get going!

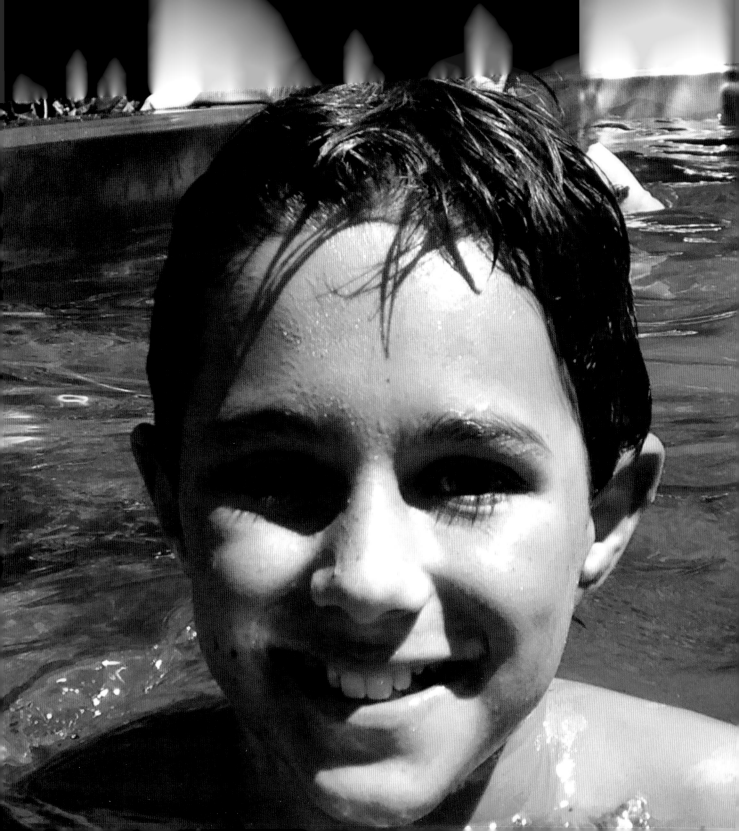

CHAPTER
TWO

The Not-So-Merry Go-Round

"Don't Deprive Them, Revive Them"

Depriving your kids of "naughty" or unhealthy foods won't work in the long term, largely because it's human nature to want what you can't have.

Think about your own adult life: you think, "alright, I am going to have an alcohol or sugar-free week" (or whatever your vice may be). You know that for your health's sake, this is a great decision and you'll feel much better for it. But how long do you last? One day, maybe two? As soon as you feel that you "can't" have something, you tend to really, really want it. And that's a typical response from an adult!

Your child has an even more exaggerated response to deprivation, because they are a kid who has not yet developed the ability to reason like an adult. So their response is entirely emotional. All they can think is "it's not fair" or "you're mean" and probably a lot more things that are even worse, unless of course you start them off with an ideal diet from birth where healthy food is their normal.

With deprivation-based strategies you are only making your life harder and theirs even unhappier. So, instead, try thinking about it as a never-ending loop, and it doesn't matter where you start, it just keeps continuing on like a not-so-merry-go-round!

The good news is that you can get off this not-so-merry-go-round at any time. And all that's required to make this change is some simple logic.

In business they call it the "80/20 Rule". By definition it means that 80 per cent of your business will come from 20 per cent of your clients. OR spend 20 per cent of your time on the clients who give you 80 per cent of your business.

But in this particular context an "80/20 Week" means:

- 80 per cent of the week = eating good food and undertaking physical activity.
- 20 per cent of the week = eating some treat foods and having some relaxation time.

With the 80/20 rule, you avoid saying a straight out "nope, you can't have that!" which is negative and deprivation-based and as such, will most likely result on a ride on that not-so-merry-go-round. Instead, the rule enables you to say "yes, you can have it every week" – which is a positive. However, as they say in marketing "conditions apply!"

In a nutshell, by implementing the 80/20 rule, you are letting kids be kids, and having the fun stuff along the way, but you're showing them how healthy food can be fun too, and cultivating positive habits that will stay with them throughout their adult life.

With the 80/20 rule comes the "80/20 Diary", which is just the same; however, it can be tailored for every child AND parent, by day, by month, by needs.

So how does it work?

If we want to make sure our kids are not on the not-so-merry-go-round, then we need to give them the tools to ensure this is the case.

The 80/20 Diary is a simple and visual way to do this. Just like their school diary, which shows them what classes they have on, what assignments are due and what tasks need to be completed, this Diary does exactly the same.

The most important part about the diary is that THEY COMPLETE IT THEMSELVES. This is because for behavioral changes to be effective, kids need to have a feeling of ownership. So this will help them feel more accountable to themselves.

In business, the best leaders allow their employees to manage their own days, tasks and plans and simply just follow up and give feedback along the way. The same can apply to your kids. Your job is to facilitate the development of the Diary, by asking questions and allowing your kids to answer for themselves. You can then follow up with them to see how they are progressing, and work with them by giving them feedback on their development.

Facilitating the start of the Diary can seem a little daunting, so here are a few steps to help you:

Step 1: Start the Conversation

An easy way to get the process started is by letting them know that you are a realist and you know that "sometimes" foods are part of their life and, therefore, something you know they will want at times. Educating the kids as to exactly why these "sometimes" foods are only to be had on an occasional basis is important so they understand why you're saying "no". It's a little like crossing the road: you have to look before you cross, so you don't get hurt. Remember, at the end of the day, it is you, the parent, who decides what goes on the shopping list, so maybe its time to have a little revisit of this list. Once there is an understanding, there is often less conflict about the situation. This is where the "conditions apply" clause kicks in. At this point you can ask them a few simple questions such as:

- "How would you feel if I took away any kind of 'sometimes' food in the house?"
- "What would it make you do?"
- "Would you like to have control over this yourself?"

These types of questions will typically elicit two feelings:

1. How it feels to have something taken away.
2. How they would behave if it was.

This then allows you to commence the first stage of them taking ownership of their own health and actions.

Step 2: Create the 80/20 Diary

This is the fun part. Here is where you get THEM to start to create their own 80/20 rules around their health. They can choose what they want to do and when, which means it's THEIR IDEA, not yours.

In the diagram on page 19 you can see an example of what a diary might look like. The hardest part of this will be around the physical aspects of the diary. If you get stuck, there are more helpful ideas in **PART 2**, which you can refer to.

Step 3: Identify the Consequences

Sir Isaac Newton's third law says that " for every action there is an equal and opposite reaction". In this situation that's called a "consequence".

Kids need boundaries and rules to help them regulate themselves, so setting up a self-managed system like this will never work unless there are consequences to the behaviors that you want to change, both positively and/or negatively.

As parents, the biggest problem we face today is *not* sticking to the consequences that we set up, if we become toothless tigers the kids know it! Rather than set them, instead, let's give them the responsibility and have them develop their own consequences.

The following chapters contain everything we learned in business, which also work at home with our kids. And trust us when we say THEY WORK! The key to success however, is unwavering consistency.

Handy
HINT ①

Let your kids choose the diary format style. Make it visual and creative so it encourages involvement.

Using different colored stickers to define activities is a starting point.

A SAMPLE 80/20 DIARY

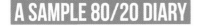

80/20 DIARY

Time	My tasks	✓
	Wake Up	
10 minutes	Do 3 x 30 second planks; or 10 x crunches; or 2 x 10 step ups on each leg; or Walk the dog around the block	
	Have breakfast | Breakfast Option: • Scrambled eggs on brown/wholemeal/sourdough toast • 1 serving of fruit (see notes for definition of one fruit serve) • 1 glass of cold water OR glass of no/ low fat milk	
	Recess Option: • 1 piece of fruit OR 4 vitaweat biscuits & cheese OR • 1 small tub of low fat yoghurt	
	Have lunch | Lunchbox Options: • Brown bread roll with ham OR cheese + lettuce and a little mayo • 1 container of chopped veggies like carrot, celery, cucumber, tomatoes • 1 lunch packet size rice crackers	
	On a non-sport afternoon, have afternoon tea. Snack Option: • Rice crackers and hummus dip • Handful of frozen grapes • 2 pieces of chocolate	
15 minutes	Fun play at home (for one) | Options: • Handball against the wall • Skipping	
	Homework time	
15 minutes	Downtime fun | Favorite TV show or computer game	
	Family dinner: Honey, Soy, Chicken with rice noodles and beans	
5 minutes	Pre-bedtime stretch | Lower back stretch	

CHAPTER
THREE

Business Principles For Raising Kids

"What Works in Business Can Work In Life"

After years of running big businesses and having to lead teams of people to great success, we had children and life turned upside-down.

We remember sitting back one day, contemplating this new job called "parenthood" and wondering "how the hell do we do it?" But then, all of a sudden, it became really clear: we do it the same way we have made hundreds of employees hugely successful! We use our proven business strategies! We realized that our decades of hard work and learning how to lead people could be directly translated to successfully raising children. The best part (for you) is that you don't have to do the years of training that we did, because we are going to give you all our key business tips.

Here are our five, just to get you started:

1. Catch them doing something right.
2. Reprimand in private not public.
3. Praise in public.
4. Set small, achievable goals.
5. Use rewards that mean something to them, not you.

TIP ①

Catch them doing something right

As human beings, one of our most natural desires in life is to "feel important". And this is even more applicable in children. We no longer live in a world filled with traditional nuclear families. In fact, there's not really any "typical" when it comes to family units nowadays, although in families where there are two parents, often both of them are working, it can be hard to ensure our children receive the recognition they need when they get things right.

Research has confirmed that rewarding good behavior is far more effective than punishing children for doing something wrong. And this is a concept that also applies to adults. Think about it: can you remember the last time you were in a job and all your boss did was tell you what was wrong? Did you feel resentful, angry, frustrated, disenchanted and disheartened? Well guess what? That's normal! So now think about how bad it must feel for a child who already feels inadequate (if they are overweight).

Of course, it's always easier to notice when things aren't right. In fact, it seems like we have become a society where the norm is to notice – or even focus – on all that is *wrong;* and this applies both at work and at home. Unfortunately, though, once we get on the "not right" train it can fast become a habit.

Think about this example: when you don't have the time and feel constantly under pressure, it's much easier to tell your children the answers to their homework questions, instead of spending the extra ten minutes encouraging them to work it out for themselves and then praising them when they do so.

When it comes to achieving a significant change in behavior, one of the keys to success is providing positive feedback. And, the more positive feedback you can provide, the more your kids will want it. Remember, children will behave based on the type of attention you give them so, if you really want them to change their behavior to become healthier (without them actually realizing that's what they're doing), then a positive reinforcement system is a great (and easy) way to make this happen.

The hardest part – as a parent – is actually doing it, and being consistent and persistent. Recognition doesn't have to be for big things; it works really well when you notice the small things too, like when you notice that they choose an apple or yogurt from the fridge instead of junk food; or when you notice they voluntarily go and do some physical activity. The "reward rather than punish" system works really well when it comes to improving health, fitness and wellness.

One easy way to provide positive feedback when you see them doing the right thing, is via a reward points system. This rewards system can be attached to the 80/20 Diary so they can see how well they commit and achieve what THEY say they will. By using this system, you are no longer the good or the bad guy, as all you are doing is following up and holding them accountable to their plan. The below diagram illustrates an example of this system.

REWARDS POINTS SYSTEM DIAGRAM

Place a sticker under each child's column, to acknowledge each time a task is achieved.

REWARDS POINTS

Task	value	mon		tues		wed		thurs		fri		w/end	
		C1	C2	C1	C2	C1	C2	C1	C2	C1	C2	C1	C2
10 Push Ups	5 points	✓		✓		✓							✓
2 pcs of fruit for brekky	10 points				✓						✓		
Walk the Dog	10 points	✓					✓						✓
No screen time	5 points				✓			✓	✓	✓			

Handy **HINT 2**

Use a small white/black board or cut out a piece of white card and stick to a wall that is in easy daily viewing areas in the house. Have a different colored marker per child attached so it's a quick and simple task to update daily.

TIP ②
Reprimand in Private

There is nothing worse than being witness to a child being publicly told off by the parents; although we've probably all been those parents at some point in time!

One thing that we can thank our parents for is that "evil eye" look we received whenever we misbehaved in public. We knew instantly if we copped the "evil eye" then we were in big trouble when we got home!

It's this private reprimand that is often considered one of the most effective forms of discipline in business. So the question is, how do we execute this strategy when it comes to improving children's health and wellness? Let's have a look at a few scenarios:

Scenario 1. You're in a hurry to get to work. The kids are running late and the house feels like its about to fall apart. You tell the kids to hurry up and get their breakfast. You go and finish getting ready for work, come out to the kitchen and see one of the kids eating chocolate or sweets as their meal. Do you:

- Scream at them to stop eating rubbish food and tell them they will get fat and punish them with no chocolate for a week?
- Walk over to them, take the sweets away and throw them in the bin. Then tell them they will have to wait until recess to eat now?

- Tell them to finish what they have in their mouth, drink their milk and pass them a piece of fruit to finish?
- None of the above, but instead scream at them saying they should know better, walk out in a huff and don't talk to them again until that night?

Scenario 2. You get home from work or from whatever chores you are doing and walk in to see the kids in the lounge with the TV blaring and them with their iPods, when it's supposed to be homework time. Do you:

- Turn the TV off, confiscate the iPods and ask them all to return to their reading or homework, then deduct this screen time from their daily allotment?
- Take their iPods, throw them in the bin and walk away?
- Yell at them for not listening to you or abiding by the rules, then ban them from any screen time for a month?
- None of the above, because you are so fed up that you don't have a clue what to do anymore?

The bottom line is, we've all been here or somewhere similar, or will be there at some point in the future. So here are some simple tips to make these sorts of scenarios a little bit easier to handle and a lot less stressful for everyone.

Using effective reprimand techniques is not

something you can achieve quickly, but once implemented a few times it can become part of the standard expectation for the household; to the point where it may actually even become self-imposed by family members. Keep in mind, we are talking about reprimanding here, not punishing. What's the difference? A "reprimand" is a formal expression of disapproval, whereas a "punishment" is to potentially treat (someone) in an unfairly harsh way.

The good news is that you don't have to always be the bad guy, because one of the keys to successfully reprimanding kids is to involve them in designing the consequences for their actions. By giving your children this level of ownership, they then have no one else to blame when it's time to be reprimanded. Of course, its not always easy and sometimes what they think is a consequence may be somewhat different to you, but just give them a chance, and with a little coaching you might be pleasantly surprised with what they come up with.

Following is a list of some great examples that our kids have come up with, and a few parent-derived options that might also fit the bill. In this example we have addressed screen time and processed foods, since they are often two of the greatest enemies for our children's health:

- "I will not play on my Playstation or play on my phone for one day"

- "I will walk the dog in the morning and afternoon"
- "I will spend 10 minutes on the trampoline instead of watching TV"
- "I will do 20 star jumps before my shower everyday for a week"

Using the 80/20 Diary, sit with the kids and get them to come up with a set of consequences for not adhering to the plan. Examples could be:

- "If I choose not to eat breakfast and buy a flavored milk on my way to school, I will forgo screen time that afternoon and, instead, will replace it with 10 star jumps, 10 push ups and 10 burpees".
- Or, "If I go over my allocated daily screen time, I will give up all screen time on the following day".

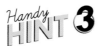

Handy
HINT 3

Make it a game and make fun. If they eat a "sometimes" food when they shouldn't then make them stop and do 20 star jumps right then and there. We call it the "20-star jump rule".

TIP 3
Praise in Public

- "Pick me, pick me!"
- "Look at me, look at what I can do!"
- "I can do it too! Look, let me have a turn!"

Do these phrases sound familiar to you? That's because during the childhood years' kids are predominantly concerned with finding their place in the world. They want nothing more than to fit in, be noticed and be liked, in a bid to make their peers and parents proud. And this applies in all aspects of their life, not just in their skills and abilities.

Considering this, when trying to make big changes to a child's health, praise can be a highly effective tool. There is so much negative media around kids being overweight and parents being responsible for the situation that it's almost become a taboo subject. The reality is, however, that childhood obesity is a massive issue and hiding from it isn't going to make it go away or any easier to deal with.

No matter how small the achievement is, praising a child in public (praising them in front of family, friends or people who are important to them) is a great way to reinforce a behavior that you want them to repeat. For example, when trying to re-educate your children about eating well and moving more, each time they pick up an apple, or they choose to walk the dog, recognize these decisions by capturing them (e.g. take a photo on your phone) and make sure that those important people know about it too.

One thing to realize about praising though is that you must only praise your kids for the traits that they have the power to change. By focusing on behaviors that are changeable you create a positive behavior loop. When a child or adult can see the results of any change they have made in their behavior, that is considered an improvement of the original behavior, which makes them want to keep doing it, as can be seen below in the Positive Behavior Diagram. Or as the scientists like to put it: By doing A it produces more of B, which in turn produces more of A.

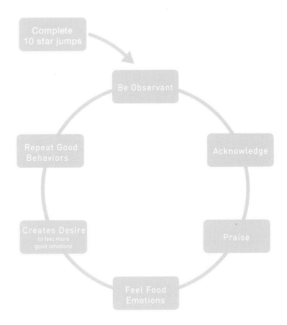

So what does this all mean?

Observe

By being conscious of being observant as much as you can, you will be in a position to see the behaviors the kids are displaying, especially in the beginning of implementing this new way.

Acknowledge

A question-style interaction is a great way to start your praise. For example, if you see them doing some sit ups, or taking the dog for a walk without being prompted by you, then acknowledge them with a question such as, "Did I just see you doing some sit ups?" or "Did you just take the dog out?"

Praise

When they reply "yes" to your acknowledging question, at that moment, right there, give them some praise. This might be in the form of a high five and/or a hug. Say "I'm proud of you", give them a big smile and a positive gesture – anything that shows them you noticed their effort, and how proud they made you feel is all they need.

Identify the Feel Good Emotions

Watch their little face light up, or they might become a bit coy; this is when you know you have hit the "feel good emotions". Enjoy it!

Create Desire to Feel More Good Emotions

These positive "feel good" emotions are addictive and, even as adults, we want more! Nothing is more important to a human being than being recognized. It makes them want more, and with wanting more their brains start to figure out more ways to get those same feelings. BINGO!

Repeat Good Behaviors

As their brains start wanting more, they will start to go looking for more ways to get you to recognize their good behaviors. And who knows? Maybe they will invent some new positive behaviors that you hadn't even thought of!

 TIP 4

Set Small, Achievable Goals

Everyone knows the old saying, "How do you eat an elephant? One bite at a time". And this couldn't be more relevant when trying to make big changes to little people's behaviors.

Setting goals that are challenging but attainable will be the fundamental piece to whether this new plan succeeds or fails. No one likes to feel their goal is so out of reach that they can't get there; if they do, they'll give up before they even start. Instead, you want the kids to think, "this is easy. I can do this!"

Setting the right goals can be the key to significant behavioral change. The goals you set should always be a SMART goal, where:

S = specific
M = measureable
A = achievable
R = relevant
T = timely

Specific: make sure the goal is specific to a behavior your child needs to change. Pin-point the major behavioral issue that will make the greatest impact, and base the goal on that. Examples could include too much screen time, not enough physical activity, over-snacking when they get home from school, or always wanting dessert.

Measureable: goals need to be measured or it's too difficult to track progress. For example, you might want your child to watch less television. Making a goal of "watching less television" is not helpful as it's difficult to monitor. Instead, a measureable goal would be "to watch no more than one hour of screen time on school days" or "to ride your bike around the block for 20 minutes on three days of the week."

Achievable: there's nothing more disheartening, disappointing or disenchanting for a child who starts off with gusto to achieve a very challenging goal but who is then unable to achieve it. It is better to start with smaller goals that are achievable, as this will boost their confidence. And then, over time, slowly make the goal more challenging. For example, if your child is currently having a packet of chips in their lunch everyday, an unachievable goal would be to have no more chips in the lunchbox – ever. Instead, you might begin by including a packet of chips in their lunchbox on just three days of the week and reduce this frequency over time.

Relevant: the goal must be relevant to the child and their behavior change. For example, there's no point making a goal to eat less chocolate when your child only eats chocolate once a week.

Timely: goals need to have a start and finish date, particularly for kids. Kids have reasonably short attention spans and their routines are usually on a weekly basis, so keeping weekly goals often works best. Setting a goal for one month or even to the end of the term can be difficult. Even for most adults, these end points can seem quite a long way away, which often sees us lose our puff and motivation before we can achieve it.

Of course, before you can work together to set goals, you as the parent, need to establish which are the most

27

important behaviors that you think need to change first. There is no point trying to change everything at once, so start with a behavior that you think is one they can change the fastest. This way they will feel a sense of achievement straight away and will be eager to try more.

This is where you as the parent or carer really need to think long and hard. Ask yourself "What is the one thing that I see every day that upsets me the most?" Is it when they don't eat breakfast and you know that they stop and buy flavored milk on the way to school? Is it because they come home from school with all their fruit still in their lunchbox? Or is it because trying to get them to do anything active is so difficult?

Maybe it's all of the above or something completely different? Whatever it is, just choose one thing; identify just one behavior that you think will be the easiest for them to modify. That's the easy part. Now you need to help them see the goal without telling them. A simple way to do this is to set them a challenge. This might be something like:

"For every 20 star jumps you do, I will do 20 star jumps and you will get 20 points. For every 100 points you earn, you can have your choice of a weekend dessert for the family."

Making it fun and including yourself in the goal shows them you care about your health too, and they see that if it's good enough for them then it's good enough for you too.

This technique will work with kids of all ages. Have them bring home their apple core or orange skin to show they ate their fruit. Start with three times a week, rather than every day, so this way they feel like they can "relax" a couple of times a week!

TIP ⑤

Use Rewards That Mean Something to Them, Not You

If someone told you that if you ate your fruit everyday at work you could go and buy your favorite book at the end of the week, would that entice you to eat more fruit? However, if someone told you that you could choose a nice restaurant to eat at if you did 20 star jumps a day would that? PROBABLY. This is even more so with kids.

They need to tell you (within reason) what rewards mean the most to them, and then as a team you can work together to establish what actions/behaviors you need to see, which will equal those rewards.

Something that is really important to remember here, is that doing something once DOES NOT equal a reward, and every reward should not be of the same value. Rewards like an extra hour of screen time might be worth 50 points, whereas having an extra treat may be worth 20 points. Using a points system is the best way to achieve continual behavioral changes, and the values that you allocate within your points system should all tie back to what real behavioral changes you want to see. This is the fun part of the process so make sure you have a laugh and a giggle along the way – especially when they throw out rewards like "Go to Bali for a vacation!"

The below diagram is of the rewards chart we use in our house. It's simple and user friendly and we have it up on a wall in our kitchen area, for everyone to see. The great thing about displaying it there is that when we have visitors, they always comment about the points – praise in public, hooray! And remember, the rewards point chart needs to be highly visible to everyone, on a daily basis.

EXAMPLE REWARDS CHART

REWARDS CHART

Task	Value	Mon		Tues		Wed		Thurs		Fri		W/end	
		C1	C2	C1	C2	C1	C2	C1	C2	C1	C2	C1	C2
I did 10 push ups	10 points	✓									✓		
I did my stretching before bed	5 points			✓				✓					
I had no screen time all day today	10 points											✓	
I didn't have any junk food today	10 points		✓							✓			
I did 10 star jumps	5 points						✓						
I walked the dog	2 points			✓									✓
I had 2 pieces of fruit at breakfast	5 points					✓				✓			
I chose a healthy after school snack	5 points											✓	
I played sport today	10 points	✓						✓		✓			

The golden rules of rewards:

- Rewards should always match the behavior change, so offer small rewards for small changes, and bigger rewards for bigger changes. Praise, hugs, a pat on the back are all free, and should be used daily to reinforce small positive changes in behaviors. Available for a small cost, you might consider items such as football cards, and then nail polish or magazines as items for the bigger, weekly rewards. The long term, bigger behavior changes (e.g. walking to/from school, three times a week for an entire term) should be acknowledged with larger rewards such as a new scooter or a shopping voucher.

- Rewards need to be relevant to the child, not to you. Agree on something that you know they'll really want to work hard for.

- Don't give rewards you already give. For example, if your child already gets to stay up late on Friday nights, don't make that the reward, as they are unlikely to work hard for it because they know they'll get it anyway.

- Give rewards at the time the positive behavior occurs. This means giving the hug or praise immediately, or buying the magazine on the agreed day, so the positive behavior is rewarded at the same time for maximum impact.

Handy **HINT 4**

Introduce a "player of the match" type of rewards system, where the best player of the week earns an extra five points, or gets to choose the family weekend treat meal. Alternatively, you can also get them to choose an exercise that a parent has to do for a day. This will make it even more fun for them and although it's not so fun for you, the truth is, it's not about you!

21 days is all it takes

There is a thing called "initial discipline". And this is the hardest type of discipline to have because, essentially, it's this type of discipline that is required in order for a specific behavior to become a permanent habit.

You need to realize that habit-forming behaviors all start with YOU. Children don't have the capacity to regulate their behaviors in the same way we can, so the habit has to start with you. If you remember our positive feedback loop (see page 25), this is where it all gets put into practice, which means this is also where the process will fail if it is not adhered to.

Once you implement the 80/20 Diary YOU MUST stay on top of it every day, for 21 days. You cannot afford the luxury of forgetting to praise and recognize or reprimand where necessary. We all know that if you forget once, you will be sending a message to your kids that the whole thing isn't really that important; and we all know that kids like to test boundaries, so you can be rest assured that they will do it here too. They will test your reactions and whether you are serious about what you say.

Be totally honest with yourself and understand that habit-forming relies first and foremost on you. If you change how you behave with them then they will, in turn, change their behaviors as well.

Key steps to forming YOUR habit:

- Put the new Diary in a place where YOU can see it all the time (even consider keeping multiple copies, if necessary).

- Focus on one goal per child, at a time – and for each child, choose the one habit that is the easiest for you to observe.

- Be overly attentive during the first week, so you don't miss anything – this means your smartphone should be out of reach for those crucial hours of home/family time.

- Acknowledge (praise or reprimand) the behavior AS SOON AS YOU SEE IT or hear about it – don't put it off until later even if you think you are too busy doing something else.

- Go to the rewards chart with your child and fill it out together.

- Watch their body language and reactions to see their "feel good emotions" and their sense of achievement (you'll feel a sense of achievement too – enjoy it!).

- As soon as you can, tell someone else about the achievement (email or phone someone together, if there's no one around to physically tell right there and then).

- REPEAT, REPEAT, REPEAT!

PART TWO

Making Physical Activity Fun And Easy

CHAPTER
FOUR

Make' Em Laugh!

"Laughter is good medicine"

Other than being good for the soul, laughing has many physical health benefits that will support a healthier and happier family life. In fact, laughter is said to:

- Boost immunity
- Lower stress hormones
- Decrease pain
- Relax muscles.

Now more than ever, as you start to make significant changes with your kids and in your home life, laughter needs to be front and center. A good reprimand followed by a little giggle shows the children that you actually want them to enjoy their life as they make these changes.

"I remember a time when saying goodnight to my son, and I stubbed my toe on a plate that was hiding under his bed. When I looked down to see what it was, I found a plate with a whole empty packet of rice crackers hiding under his bed. I was exhausted and not in the mood, so felt my temper starting to raise its ugly head – not just for the fact that my

toe hurt, or at the thought we may have a pending cockroach plague from all the food on the floor, but also because he hid it. As I started to reprimand him, his little face reflected his own disappointment that he'd upset me, to which I asked him to tell me why he thought I was upset. He told me, and then followed it up with 20 push ups. But to make it fun, I joined in and we turned it into a competition to see who could get them done first. By the end of it he was laughing at me because I lost; however, he also understood what not to do next time he felt like a midnight snack!"

Nicole Monteforte

Obviously, laughter can't be forced but there are many ways to encourage it. Try a few of these gag busters next time you feel the tension brewing after a reprimand, or when you can see the loath in their eyes when you enforce the "20-star jump rule":

- Yoga pose holds: One person "creates" a yoga pose and everyone else has to copy that pose. The person who can stay in that position the longest (without falling over) earns 10 points.
- Funny face-off: Whoever can pull off the best funny face, wins! Score each face out of 10 and the one who earns the most points, wins!
- Planking competition: Whoever can hold themselves the longest in the "plank" position without collapsing to the ground earns 10 points.
- The "Hahaha Off": Get the whole family lying down on the ground on their back with each person's head resting on the tummy of another family member. One person starts by doing a short fake "ha ha ha" laugh, and you see how long it takes before everyone is actually laughing so hard they can't stop.

CHAPTER FIVE

Physical Activity Made Easy... At Home

"Make Movement Fun and It Won't Ever Seem Like A Chore Again"

Many parents believe that in order to get your kids active, you have to leave the house, or invest huge amounts of effort or money. But this simply isn't true.

After a busy day the last thing most parents want, is to have to put in more effort to make sure their kids do some sort of physical activity. If your children are already involved with extra curricular or after school sports, then you'll only need to think about how they can be active on the days they don't have sport. Or, if your kids aren't involved in organized sport already then what can you do?

Trust us, we know the dilemma of having to get kids out from under your feet so you can cook, unpack lunchboxes, answer emails, make phone calls or do whatever else needs to be done in order to manage your life, but yet still steer them away from sedentary activities.

After much trial and error, as well as persistence (and the realization that getting them started is always the hardest part of this process), we have compiled a list of some of our all-time favorite activity ideas, which have all worked a treat with our own kids.

Plus, we've made it even easier for you by dividing them into categories such as "After School" and "Weekend" activities. And obviously, on the weekends there is (hopefully) a little more time available for you to join in and be involved (which will go a long way to ensuring you look after your health as well).

Once you've passed the challenge of "getting started", the kids will love the activities so much that you'll be able to leave them to entertain themselves whilst also feeling assured that they are in "energy out" mode and, therefore, living a healthier life!

If you don't have a backyard, don't worry! There are many options in our lists that do not require one. Also, there are many options that can be done in any space, whether it's a front lawn, garage, lounge room, the driveway of your apartment, or wherever. Many of the listed activities can be adapted to all kinds of property situations.

Note: Although we've divided the activity options into "After School" and "Weekend" categories, in reality you can do most of them at any time of any day during the week or weekend.

Activity Option 1. Balloon Tennis

Where to play: Indoors or in small spaces.

How many people: Ideal for one or more children.

What you'll need: A few balloons and a medium-sized floor space (preferably on a mat).

Set up: Set up a "net" using a skipping rope or a few books in a straight line, placed in the middle of the space you're playing in. One half of the players stay on one side of the net, and the other half play on the other side. As a parent/carer you can be a player in the game or you can choose to be the umpire.

How to play: Like regular tennis, players hit the balloon to and fro over the net. The aim is to keep the balloon in the air and avoid letting it touch the ground.

If it does touch, all the players on the other side of the net to where the balloon touched the ground will each score a point. If it is a player of one, the idea is to score no points for as long as possible.

Why it's so good: It encourages movement, flexibility and incorporates every muscle in the body.

Caution: Remove any dangerous furniture or fragile breakables from within or around the playing space. The game is designed to be fun, not destructive.

Activity Option 2. Poison Ball

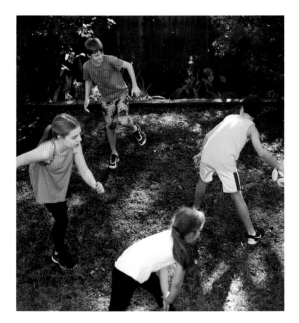

Where to play: Best played outside.

How many people: Two or more people.

What you'll need: A small to medium size soft ball.

How to play: One person has the ball and tries to get somebody else "out" by throwing the ball at the legs of all other players. Whenever the ball touches someone's legs, that person is "out" and it then becomes their turn to throw the ball at the other players.

Why it's so good: The kids will be laughing and running around for hours. But be warned, kids love parents getting involved in this game so they can get you "out". Not only will this game keep your kids fit, but you'll get your heart rate up too!

Activity Option 3. Basketball

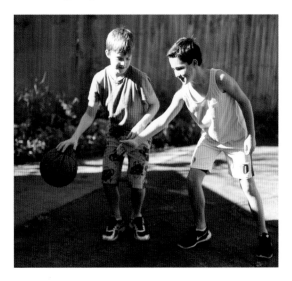

Where to play: Indoors or outdoors.

How many people: One or more.

What you'll need: A small basketball ring and a basketball that fits through the ring.

Set up: Set up one of those small indoor basketball rings. Designate a spot where each team needs to shoot from; ideally, choose an area that allows players to run to a certain turning point, and back again. Remember – the longer the running distance, the better.

How to play: Each participant has 10 attempts to shoot a goal from pre-designated spots. You need to time how long it takes each person, and the person who does it in the fastest time, wins. Then, over time, the goal should be to reduce the time it takes to score the 10 baskets. As an alternative, you can work against the clock and see how many goals can be achieved in a set amount of time. In this instance, the winner will be the person with the most number of goals scored in that set time.

Why it's so good: Shooting will strengthen the upper body and help the core muscles. It will enhance hand-eye coordination and by having them focus on gaining a faster time or more goals, they will typically begin running rather than walking, during this activity.

Activity Option 4. Elastics (also sometimes called "French Skipping")

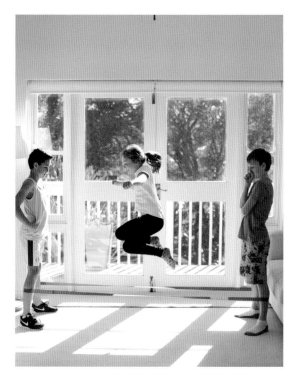

Where to play: In an open space that will accommodate the stretched out elastic and where people can freely jump up and down.

How many people: To play properly, you'd traditionally need a minimum of four players, but you could get away with only three and a bin (or if absolutely necessary, one person and three heavy chairs!).

What you'll need: A *really* long piece of knickers elastic – the kind that's about 5mm wide. The ideal size for playing with four people would be around 3m.

Set up: Stretch the elastic around the ankles of three players (or your chosen heavy inanimate objects if you're a bit short on players).

How to play: The one remaining player then performs a series of jumping moves to ensure that after each manoeuvre their feet land in specific positions. These positions may include:

- both feet under the elastic
- both feet on top of the elastic
- one on top, one under
- one foot on top, one foot under, and then swap feet before moving to the next stretch of elastic (known as 'swapsies')

After successfully completing a round of all the jump types above, the height of the elastic is raised from the ankles (increasing the challenge/difficulty of the jumps) to 'kneesies', then 'thighsies' before 'waistsies' and then the real challenge, which is 'chesties'.

If the current player fails to execute a jump successfully, then their turn is over and play is passed to one of the people who are holding the elastic (or awaiting players if there are more than four people involved). The goal is for each player to try and progress further than the others.

Why it's so good: Although traditionally a girl's game, elastics can really sort the men from the boys (so to speak). Precision jumping skills and supreme concentration is required in order to excel at this game. Any activity where your feet leave the ground is guaranteed to significantly increase your heart rate, which means that it will enhance your cardio fitness and all the benefits that go along with this.

Activity Option 5. Hopscotch

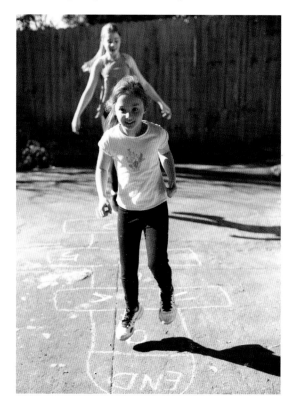

Where to play: All you need is a flat surface (I would recommend the footpath as it can get messy) and some chalk.

How many people: Ideal for one or more children.

What you'll need: Nothing more than chalk, a stone and good balance.

Set up: Draw as many "single" and "double jump" squares as you want. Remember, the longer the hopscotch board the better it is for everyone's fitness. Number each square.

How to play: Standing in front of square one, participants throw the stone so it lands on a square. They must then hop on every square until they get to the one with the stone on it. They need to stop and (if on one foot, stay on one foot) bend over and pick up the stone before continuing on to the end. At the end they must turn around and hop back to the start.

Why it's so good: Great for balance. Jumping or hopping significantly increases your heart rate and aids your cardiovascular system. So this game is great for weight loss, toning and general fitness.

Activity Option 6. Balance a Book on Your Head

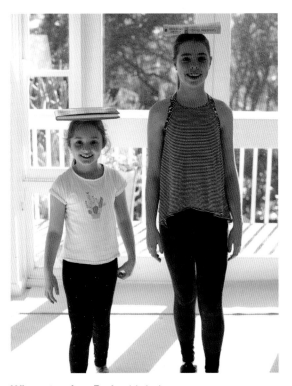

Where to play: Preferably indoors.

How many people: The beauty of this game is that it can be played by one person or as many as you want.

What you'll need: A good solid book. Remember, if the book falls you could slightly damage it, so don't use a favorite. It needs to have some weight but nothing too heavy.

Set up: Stand at a designated starting place, and balance a book on top of the head.

How to play: Walk to a designated point, turn around and then come back to the starting point. Running is not allowed and if the book falls off they must stop and place the book back on their head before continuing. Each person must complete the course once. Alternatively, have two to four people race against each other.

Why it's so good: This enforces good posture, which means that the kids have to activate their core muscles; and a stronger core means a stronger structure.

Activity Option 7. Wheelbarrow Races

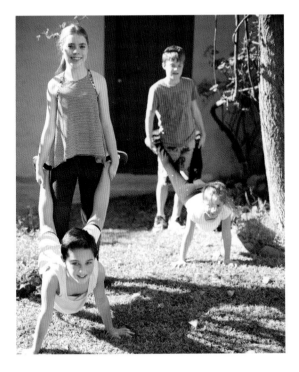

Where to play: Outside, on a flat grassed area.

How many people: You need a minimum of two people. The game is ideal with groups of four, six or eight people.

What you'll need: Nothing but a little bit of upper body strength.

Set up: One person starts by kneeling on their hands and knees on the grass. The other person then lifts up their legs, so they become the "wheelbarrow".

How to play: Kids divide into teams of two, with one person in each team dropping down on the ground, to their hands and knees. The other person in the team lifts up their legs so their weight rests through their hands (like a handstand). They must then walk on their hands until they reach the end of the course. Once there, the participants switch places to walk back.

Why it's so good: Improves upper body strength and challenges the core muscles.

41

Activity Option 8. Duck, Duck Goose (in a group)

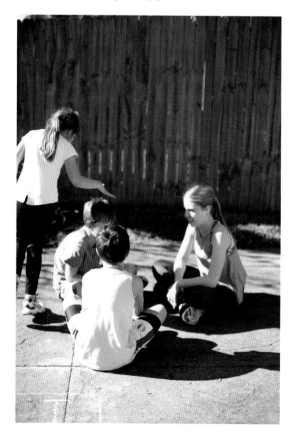

How to play: One person is named "it", and walks around the outside of the circle. As they walk around, they tap people's heads and say whether they are a "duck" or a "goose". Once someone is named a "goose" they must get up to their feet and chase "it" around the outside of the circle. The goal is for the "goose" to tap the "it" person before "it" runs the complete circle and sits down in the goose's space. If the goose is not able to do this, they become "it" for the next round and play continues. If they do tap the "it" person, then that person tagged has to sit in the center of the circle. The goose then becomes "it" for the next round. The person in the middle cannot leave until another person is tagged and only then, are they replaced in the middle.

Why it's so good: It's a great game for creating a good social environment for a group of kids. It will also get the kids running (actually sprinting) a fair bit too, so it has a good cardiovascular component.

Where to play: Outside. You could use a medium to large size backyard or a local park.

How many people: This game is best when you have 10 or more people in the group or circle. Less than 10 and the circle is too small.

Set up: Players sit down in a circle facing each other.

Activity Option 9. 'What's the Time Mr. Wolf?'

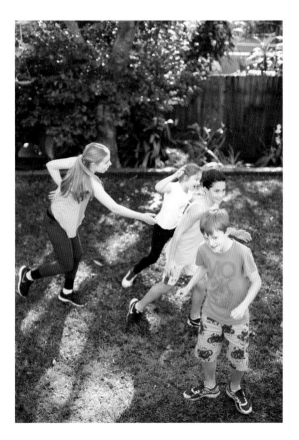

How to play: The other players shout out "What's the time Mr. Wolf?" Mr. Wolf must then respond with an answer of "1 o'clock" or "2 o'clock" or, in fact, any number "o'clock" between 1 and 12. The players must then take that number of steps in the direction of Mr. Wolf. Once the players get close enough to Mr. Wolf, Mr. Wolf can reply to the question with the words "Dinner time!" instead of an "o'clock" answer, in which case he chases the other players with the goal to catch someone. That caught person will now become Mr. Wolf for the next round.

Why it's so good: Similar to "Duck, Duck, Goose" this game has a good cardiovascular component. But most importantly, it will have them smiling and laughing while participating.

Where to play: In a backyard or open space.

How many people: Two or more.

Set up: One person stands at one end of the backyard with their eyes covered and their back towards the other players. They are "Mr. Wolf".

43

Activity Option 10. Backyard Soccer

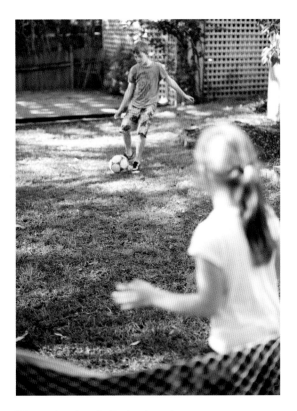

Where to play: In the backyard.

How many people: The beauty of this game is that you can play with as little as two people, or as many as 20.

- With a small group: Set up one soccer goal (if you don't have a soccer goal, you can place two items of clothing on the ground as goal posts).

Play "shoot outs" where whoever scores the most goals, wins.

- With a large group: Set up two sets of goals and play a proper game of soccer.

Set up: You don't need a large backyard for this but if you do have some space, set up a goal post using one or two chairs.

How to play: You can play a mini game of soccer, or just even take shots at goals. Parents can be the goalies and try and stop the kids' shots from getting through.

If you have limited space available, try balancing/ kicking drills instead. These could include challenges such as:

- How many times can you kick the ball on one foot before it touches the ground?
- How many times can you kick the ball when you use alternating legs?

Why it's so good: This game doesn't just promote cardiovascular fitness, it will also assist in developing a child's gross motor skills, particularly in their lower body when kicking and controlling the ball.

CHAPTER
SIX

Physical Activity Made Easy... Outdoors

"Getting Out and About Has Never Been Easier – Or More Fun!"

Whether your job is to manage the house or sell stocks and bonds, it doesn't matter, because when Friday comes around we are typically filled with relief that we can have a rest! But of course, guess what? That usually never happens when you have kids, so you have to plan ahead to ensure that your weekend allows the family to get out together and have some fun.

"I remember feeling so much anxiety leading up to a busy weekend where I had four kids to entertain. Fortunately, planned extracurricular sport took up a few hours on Saturday mornings; however, it was that dreaded thought of "what am I going to do to entertain them after sport" that plagued my mind in the wee hours of the night.

With a little pre-planning though, the weekends ended up being full of activities such as trampolining, basketball competitions, sandcastle building at the beach, scooter races, flower collecting, street walks and some plain old floor wrestling. By Sunday nights the kids were so exhausted (as were we) that they were all begging to go to bed early. In fact, the three-

year-old often didn't even make it to bed before he nodded off!" Says Shane

Now it sounds hard work but in all honesty the hard work comes when you have nothing to do and they are bored and whining at you all weekend!

Pre-planning your weekends is actually not as daunting as it may sound; however, it does require a bit of effort to carry it off. But, once you learn the tricks, your weekends will be filled with activities but also the down time that you deserve (and probably need).

So here are a few activities, which always proved popular in my household. Feel free to adapt them to suit your environment, equipment and your kids' abilities and likes/dislikes. Hopefully they'll also inspire your own ideas for new activities.

Activity Option 1. Mini Kids' Triathlon

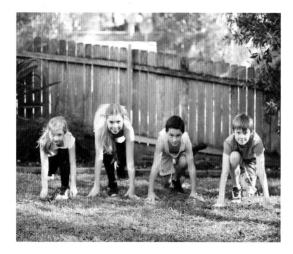

Where to play: Ideally a local park, where there's plenty of space. Other options could include the footpath in your street or the hallway (if you have one) in your house. All you need to do is change the activity options to cater for the space you have access to.

How many people: Minimum of four... and parents, get your runners on for this one!

What you'll need: This will depend on what sports you want to incorporate into the mini triathlon. Examples are bikes, soccer balls or footballs. However you can also follow the 'How to play' below which requires no additional equipment:

Set up: Players divide into teams of two. Identify the triathlon course (e.g. use a start and an end point, such as two trees, and that becomes your course).

How to play:

First leg: Race walk (this provides a little more fun than a straight run).

Second leg: Complete 10 sit ups.

Third leg: Hopping race.

Why it's so good: The activity options for this game are limited only by your imagination. Combining three different activities will give them a great workout, whilst also having a huge amount of fun!

Activity Option 2. Frisbee competition

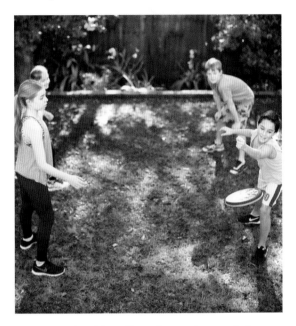

Where to play: You will need a good amount of space to run around, so a local park is an ideal venue.

How many people: Minimum of two people.

What you'll need: A Frisbee and nothing else.

Set up: Work out the distance that each player must stand from the other players.

How to play: A great little game is to come up with a word, such as "donkey" or even "Frisbee". The goal of the game is to NOT drop the Frisbee, or to make the other players drop it. When a player drops the Frisbee, they receive a letter (e.g. "D" as in "donkey"). And every time they drop the Frisbee they receive another letter. The first player to get the whole word ("donkey" or "Frisbee") loses.

Why it's so good: This will help them develop their hand-eye coordination, as well as challenge their basic gross motor skills.

Activity Option 3. Hide and Seek

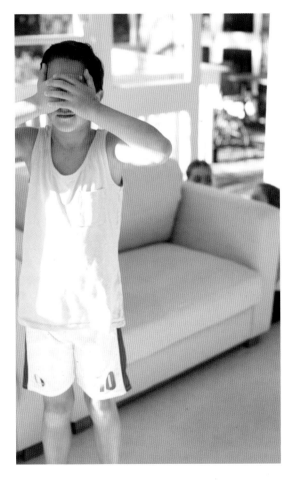

Where to play: Anywhere. This is a game that can be played both inside and outdoors.

How many people: A minimum of three people are needed, but the more the better.

What you'll need: Preferably a large space with numerous places to hide.

Set up: IMPORTANT RULE – You must set the boundaries for the game before starting. Be aware of any roads or any areas that you wouldn't feel comfortable letting the kids go to.

How to play: One person covers their eyes and counts up to 20 or 50. The rest of the players run away to find a hiding spot. Once someone has been found, they help the seeker find the other players. Once everyone has been found, it's the player who was found first who now becomes the seeker.

Why it's so good: This game is a great option to play in your home when the weather outside is poor.

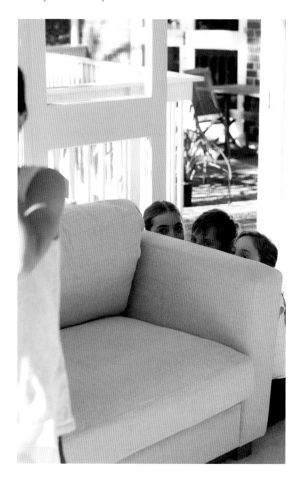

48

Activity Option 4. Hide a ball/item competition

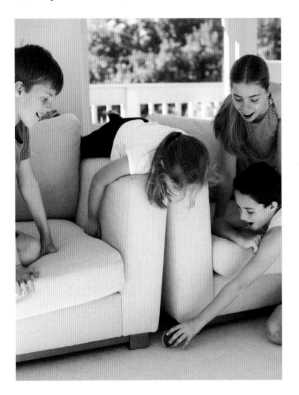

Where to play: This is another game that can be played anywhere. This one is a great game to play indoors when the weather outside is nasty.

How many people: Two or more, plus one person to hide the item.

What you'll need: Any medium size item such as a ball, a clothing item, a rope or a toy.

Set up: Designate one part of the house where the "seekers" can wait while the item is hidden. One person then goes and hides the item somewhere in the house. **Note:** Parents should establish the boundaries or any areas in the house that cannot be used as hiding places. Give the "hider" 1-minute to hide the item.

How to play: To make this game energetic, you must include a time limit to find the item. You can change the time limit based on the size of your house and/or number of players. I would suggest a time limit of one to three minutes. Make it difficult for them to find or make the time short, and it will mean the kids will be running around frantically trying to find the item.

Why it's so good: Just like most adults, kids love challenges! So adding a time limit to this game completely changes how the kids feel about playing it. Running to find the item will give the kids a great cardio workout, plus finding the item will give them a distinct sense of achievement.

CHAPTER
SEVEN

Kids and Resistance Training

"Keep Them Interested with Moderation and Variety"

A strong body is important for everyone including kids. Having been around gyms and fitness for over 20 years, we have pretty much seen it all when it comes to kids and working out.

According to the Mayo Clinic children can begin strength exercises as early as eight years of age and although weight training exercises are not recommended for children under the age of 12, there are some exercises that use resistance, which can help children build muscle and stay lean. Ideally, for muscle building, children's exercises should focus on bodyweight movements, such as those detailed opposite, as well as the use of resistance bands.

'With a 12-year-old son and a 13-year-old dancer in my house, being strong and flexible is important. So the big issue is "how do I teach them what is best for their body, without doing anything that could damage their growing ligaments?" This dilemma forced me to really think about what to do and what not to do, and the result is the following very simple strength routine, which can be undertaken pretty much anywhere, at any time." Said Nic

A FEW TIPS BEFORE YOU START

All of the workout options are set around the concept of the body's basic movement patterns, which we predominately use in our regular day-to-day lives.

Basic Movement	Day-to-Day Example
Squat	Sitting
Lunge	Walking up stairs
Push	Pushing a pram or opening a door
Pull	Opening/closing a car door
Bend	Picking up clothes from the floor
Twist	Putting on your seatbelt

The benefit for anyone incorporating these movement patterns into their workout is that it allows you to challenge a large number of your big muscles, which burn more calories (increasing the "energy out"). It also supports how your body moves in daily life.

When you go to sit down, the movement is a squat. When you walk, your legs move in a lunge movement. Opening or closing a door uses the push and pull movement. Your kids should do exercises that improve the strength required for them to undertake basic body movement patterns.

What you'll need:

- Comfortable (but not too loose) clothing.
- Comfortable and supportive running shoes.
- Towel.

The number one rule when it comes to exercise is:

- You need to drink 1 x 500ml water bottle for each 30 minutes of working out.

Basic principles for each 30-minute workout:

- Perform the exercise at a speed of 3 seconds on the up phase of the exercise, and 3 seconds on the down phase.
- For each exercise complete 3 sets of 10 repetitions.
- Between each exercise set, have a 1-minute rest (no longer).

Exercise terminology/definitions:

- A "set" is the completion of a certain number of the relevant exercise (e.g. "complete 3 sets of the exercise").
- A "repetition" (also known as a "rep") is one complete movement of the exercise (e.g. "complete 12 reps to do 1 set").

Progressing (or advancing) an exercise:

When starting an exercise use these below rules before progressing to the next level.

Rule 1: Start by performing 8 reps (complete movements of the exercise).

Rule 2: Try and perform 1 extra rep of the exercise, every day.

Rule 3: Once you can perform 15 reps of the exercise, the next day you can progress the exercise and go back to completing 8 reps.

THE EXERCISES

Exercise 1. Push Ups (push movement)

What it does: Push ups are bodyweight exercises that strengthen the core, shoulders, chest and triceps.

How to do it: Place your hands on the floor. They should be in line with your shoulders (see photos). With your legs straight and feet together, drop your body down towards the floor until your chest almost touches the floor.

How many to do: As it is a "bodyweight" exercise, you can try and complete as many push ups as possible. Start with 8 reps and then the following day add 1 more. The next day add another. And so on.

Progression: Most kids start off with a modified push up, which are done on the knees, rather than the toes.

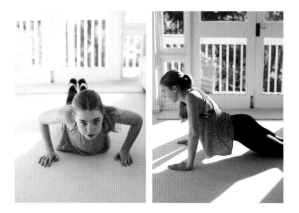

Once they become strong enough, they can work towards performing a more advanced version (on the toes), as shown below.

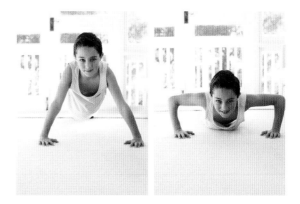

Exercise 2. Pull Ups (pull movement)

What it does: Pull ups use a child's bodyweight to target the biceps and back muscles.

Caution: Children performing pull ups should always train with the supervision of an adult.

How to do it: Find a bar or possibly a fence and hanging on with your hands, drop your body under the bar/fence. Start with your legs bent at a 90-degree angle and pull yourself up towards the bar or fence until your chest almost touches.

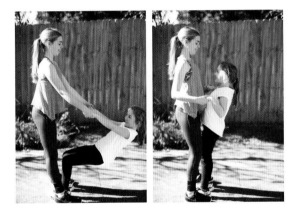

How many to do: Again, start with completing 8 repetitions and work your way from there. Once you get to 15, progress to the below option.

Progression: To increase the difficulty of the exercise, straighten your legs throughout the movement.

Exercise 3. Sit Ups / Crunches (bend movement)

What it does: This exercise strengthens the abdominal muscles, which are also known as the "core" muscles.

Caution: When performing a sit up (also called a "crunch") children should focus on keeping their feet flat on the ground throughout the complete movement.

How to do it: When performing a sit up or a crunch, the arms should remain straight throughout the whole exercise. Place the hands on the legs, and as the sit up is performed, slide the hands up the legs until you touch your kneecaps.

For a more advanced exercise, place hands at the side of your head slightly touching ears. Sit up all the way until your upper body reaches your thighs then lower yourself slowly counting to 5 on the way down.

Caution: Make sure that your neck stays in a straight line with your back throughout the exercise.

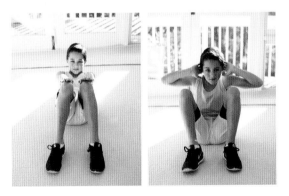

How many to do: Start with at least 10 to 12 reps and try to increase this number to 20 before progressing.

53

Exercise 4. Sit Ups Twist (bend/twist)

What it does: This exercise strengthens the abdominal muscles.

Caution: Avoid straining the neck by keeping it in a neutral position. You can do this by imagining that you are holding a small tennis ball underneath your chin.

How to do it: Lying on the floor. Back flat. Bend your legs as much as possible (see image). Raise your upper body slightly off the ground. From this position, twist your upper body sideways until you can 'tap' your heel with your fingers. Repeat this movement on the other side of your body.

How many to do: Again, the same principle applies. Start with 10 to 12 reps. Increase by 1 per day until you can complete 20 repetitions.

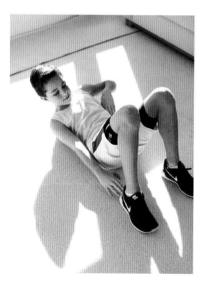

Exercise 5. Lunges

What it does: Strengthens the quadriceps, hamstrings and glutes.

How to do it: Stand with the right foot straddled in front of the body. Placing a chair next to you is handy to help with balance. Your back foot should be facing forward with the heel in the upward position. Bend both knees and drop down so that legs form a 90-degree angle. The knee on the front leg should not go past the toe. Return to the top and repeat.

How many to do: 10 to 12 repetitions.

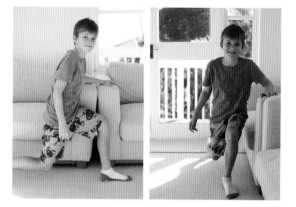

Progression: Again, remove the chair and perform the same exercise. This makes the movement significantly tougher.

Exercise 6. Squats (squat movement)

What it does: Strengthens the major muscles in the legs (i.e. glutes, quadriceps and hamstrings) and improves balance. Squats for kids are executed using bodyweight only. Proper technique will deliver the best and safest results.

How to do it: To begin a squat, stand with the feet a little wider than hip-width apart. Extend the arms out in front of the body to ensure balance and control of the movement. Keep the chest up, and sit back as if you're about to take a seat in a chair. The knees should stay behind the toes as the child squats about halfway down. Come back to start and repeat.

How many to do: 10 to 12 repetitions.

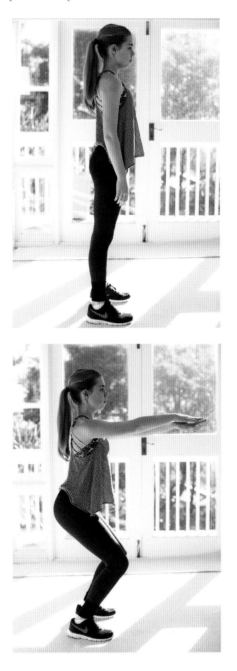

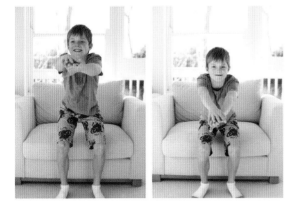

Progression: Take the chair away and perform the same exercise without the chair. Look to drop your body a little bit lower than what the chair would allow you to go.

CHAPTER
EIGHT

Let's Get Stretchy

"A Little Bit of Stretch Can Last A Lifetime"

Kids are traditionally far more flexible than adults, however as they hit their teenage years, if they don't continue to make use of their flexibility it starts to rapidly diminish. Add to this the fact that kids are spending more time on computers and devices, stretching becomes an even more important activity. After all, it is one of the best solutions to combatting the stress and poor posture that this lifestyle often encourages.

Even though there are many ways to warm up and cool down before and after exercise, stretching is an important part of both those processes. Staying flexible has significant long term health benefits, not to mention the calming effect it can have on the body.

The type of stretches that we've provided in this chapter, are known as static stretches. This is because you hold the end position for approximately 20 seconds. Benefits of static stretching include:

1. Reduction in risk of muscle joint injury
2. Increased flexibility
3. Joint range and motion
4. Increased blood flow to the muscles.

Stopping and taking five minutes to stretch is often NOT the most appealing activity for an adult, let alone a child, so to boost its appeal focus on the fun factor (as well as the points you allocate to the activity). Here are a few simple fun ways you can get the kids to stretch regularly:

- Make it a daily family activity that is done right before dinner. Choose three stretches from our options below, and get every family member involved and holding each stretch for 1-minute.
- With smaller kids make stretching an animal game. Change the names of some of the stretches to reflect different types of animals. You could say something like "stretch like a cat" or "make yourself long like a snake".
- Print out one stretch and put in on the back of the front door. Every time someone leaves the house they have to hold that stretch for 45 seconds before they leave.

Stretch 1: Calf Stretch

How to: Leaning against a wall, take a large step backwards with one leg. While keeping your back straight, push the heel on the back leg down towards the floor. The goal is to have the complete sole of the foot on the floor. Breathe in and out for 10 seconds. Hold this position for 3 rounds of breathing. Repeat these instructions with the other leg.

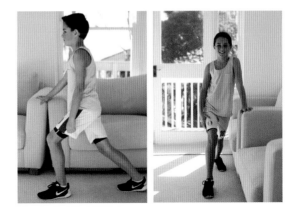

Stretch 2: Hamstring Stretch

How to: Sitting on the floor, up tall with a straight spine, extend the right leg out in front of you. Bend your left leg and place your left foot against the inside of your upper right thigh. Place both arms onto the right leg and keeping both arms straight, slowly slide them down the extended leg. Breathe in and out for 10 seconds. Hold this position for 3 rounds of breathing. Repeat these instructions with the left leg.

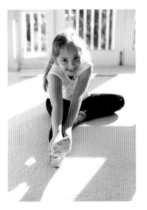

Stretch 3: Quadricep Stretch

How to: Standing next to a wall or chair for balance, bend you right knee so that your foot is close to your bottom. With your right hand grab your right ankle. Breathe in and out for 10 seconds, then release the right leg. Repeat these instructions with the left leg. Repeat twice on each leg.

Stretch 4: Hip Stretch

How to: Standing up feet together hands above your head in prayer position, take one large step back. With your back leg remaining straight, push back heel down to the ground. Whilst completing this exercise, your eyes should be looking at the top of your fingertips. Hold for 10 seconds and repeat on alternate leg.

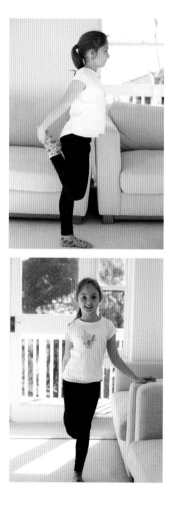

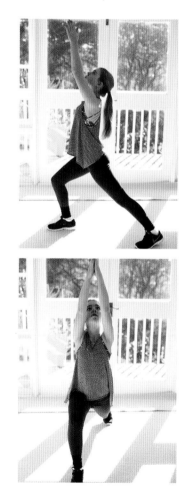

Stretch 5: Mid Back Stretch

How to: Kneel on all fours. As you breathe in, arch your back up to the sky and as you breath out, lower the arch by pushing your abdominals to the ground, so your back is in a reverse arch. Repeat this action 4 times.

Stretch 6: Lower Back Stretch

How to: Lie on your back with your arms stretched out straight on either side of your body. Bring your knees up into the V position and roll them over to one side whilst turning your head in the opposite direction. Hold for 10 seconds and roll legs over to the other side and hold again. Concentrate on breathing deeply throughout.

Caution: Be mindful of your core throughout this exercise. To ensure your back is kept strong and straight, suck your belly button down into the floor with every movement.

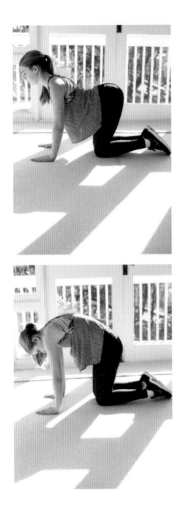

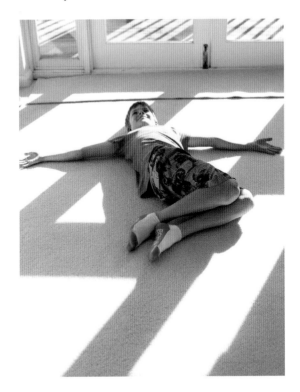

Stretch 7: Tricep Stretch

How to: Raise one arm above your head and bend the elbow so the palm of your hand is resting against the top of your spine, as if you are trying to scratch the middle part of your back.

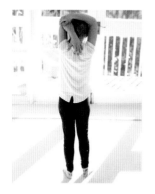

Stretch 8: Shoulder Stretch

How to: Standing next to a wall place the palm of your hand flat on the wall. Slowly rotate your feet so that your body is facing away from the wall and your bottom is now facing the wall. Hold for 10 seconds and repeat on other arm.

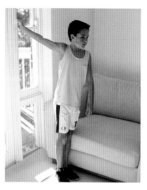

Stretch 9: Pectoral Stretch

How to: Stand next to a wall and place your arm along the wall at shoulder height. Move your upper body forwards and slowly rotate away from the wall until you feel a stretch in your chest. Hold for 10 seconds and repeat on other arm. Hold this position for 3 rounds of breathing.

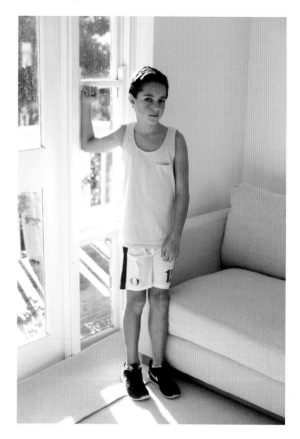

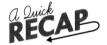

For a healthier and happier family and future, the key messages with regards to physical activity are:

- Plan regular family activities that revolve around physical activity: go for a walk, play in the park, toss a baseball, or take the family pet for a tour of the neighborhood.
- Set limits for the amount of television that can be watched, and include computer and video game time in these limits.
- Focus on introducing small, gradual changes, as little changes help to build life-long healthy habits.
- Be supportive and sensitive. Remember that everyday is a work in progress and that effort matters – especially when it comes to losing weight or maintaining weight loss, which can feel like a constant struggle.

Everyone in the family needs to get moving, and keep moving regularly!

CHAPTER EIGHT *Let's Get Stretchy*

PART THREE

Food And Nutrition – Where To Start

A WORD FROM OUR NUTRITIONIST, JAIME ROSE CHAMBERS

As a qualified and practising dietitian, I have spent close to a decade of my career focusing on children's nutritional issues, ranging from fussy eaters, food allergies and intolerances, big appetites, little appetites, food aversions, overweight, inactivity and many more. These days, when it comes to their kids' nutrition, parents are facing more challenges than ever, despite the overwhelming amount of information available to them. The common denominator is that they all want the best for their kids, and this includes a healthy diet and great nutrition.

Children today live in a very different nutritional environment compared to when I was a child. These days, they are constantly exposed to a barrage of advertising on TV and in the supermarkets for new, fun and exciting packaged foods. Once upon a time, kids were naturally active, always playing in the streets, walking or biking to school, and running around all lunchtime. Nowadays, children are far less active; there is often limited space to run around and if they're living in the city or the crowded suburbs, then there's usually no backyard to play in. And it's difficult for parents to let children wander to the local park, as they are often concerned for their safety.

We see busy parents racing from one place to the next, piling the kids into and out of the car, driving everywhere because there's not enough time to walk there. Then, throw in a child or two who are fussy eaters, and all of a sudden parents find themselves having to make multiple meals in the evening, just to avoid the nagging for more food or the cries of "I'm still hungry" – it's no surprise that life can feel very rushed for everyone involved, which can result in parents feeling defeated, deflated and a bit lost when it comes to feeding the family.

The aim of the following nutrition chapter is, therefore, to very simply outline the general nutritional guidelines for kids, and what that looks like in practical terms. I've also included some helpful tips to deal with a range of different nutrition and food-based issues, as well as some easy, tried and tested, nutritious recipes that you and your kids are bound to enjoy.

CHAPTER
NINE

Nutrition Basics For Kids

"Simple Things Can Make Life Easy"

Remember when your daily food intake consisted of cornflakes, an apple, a cheese sandwich, maybe a packet of crisps, meat and three veg, and if you were lucky, maybe a bowl of vanilla ice cream?

Nowadays is a different story, when it comes to diet things have changed. Should you give them juice or shouldn't you? Which bread is the right bread? How are we ever supposed to know what is right and what is wrong and what is the best for our little ones, when everyday there is a magnitude of information being thrown at us. From countless sources we are being told something different – not to mention, the constant and relentless advertising campaigns promoting unhealthy and high in sugar snack foods at every possible opportunity.

Feeding your kids and keeping them happy and healthy can feel like a real nutritional minefield to manoeuvre, and a scary one at that.

The simplest thing you can do is stick to the 80/20 rule.

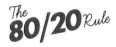

A Refresher

- *80 per cent of the week = eating good food and undertaking physical activity*
- *20 per cent of the week = eating some treat foods and having some relaxation time.*
  (Refer back to Chapter 2 for a full recap about the 80/20 rule.)

The following recipes and snacks are very easy to prepare, and taste great. You might want to add some fun to some of the snacks to make them even more visually enticing until your kids get used to eating them.

Smart Snacking

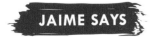

"One of the most common complaints I hear from parents is that their kids are driving them crazy, by endlessly complaining about being hungry, and getting under their feet or milling around in the kitchen between meals. This is often just a bad habit or a result of them feeling bored. So, by ensuring your kids' snacks are well structured you'll be able to get them to the next main meal with a lot less frustration.

Unfortunately, these days most snack bars and packaged foods that go into lunchboxes are far from nutritious, and tend to put a big nutritional hole in our kids' diet. Instead of providing the energy kids need to perform, unhealthy and processed snacks are more likely to cause blood sugar spikes and crashes leaving them hungry in an hour of eating. The snacks we suggest are packed with the nutritious stuff kids need to get through sports, school classes and homework, and to perform on a daily basis.

The golden rule with snacks is that they need to be a combination of a good quality carbohydrate and some protein or fats. Complex carbohydrates are the only nutrient that lift our blood sugar levels and take away that feeling of hunger. It's like putting petrol in a car and the red light turning off. These complex carbohydrates, when combined with protein or fat, will sustain the kids for longer, resulting in less tugging on your shirt between meals, asking "whheeeeeen will dinner be ready?"

The problem though, is that these days those carbohydrates have become a lot less "complex". They are more processed than ever and when you couple this with picky, fussy eaters who won't touch the brown bread or the stuff with the seedy bits in it, it makes life tough. Think white bread with Vegemite, Milo or LCM Bars – these snacks have almost no nutritional value as there's no fiber, vitamins, minerals, slow release carbohydrates or protein.

65

So here's my list of the perfect snack combinations. How creative you are with these snacks, what foods you keep available in your home, and the level of involvement your kids have in putting their snack together will all determine the success you have in getting them to eat and enjoy them:

- Small bowl of fruit salad with a dollop of yogurt
- 4 wholegrain crackers with cheese
- Veggie sticks and hummus
- Fruit kebab with yogurt dipping sauce
- 40 g (1.4 oz) cubed cheese with half a chopped apple
- 30 g (1 oz) of wheat flakes with light milk and 1 teaspoon of honey
- 1 slice of brown toast with avocado
- 1 small tub of low fat yogurt and a handful of berries
- 4 pieces of dried fruit and 10 nuts
- 2 big celery sticks filled with peanut butter
- 1, 20–30 g (1 oz) piece of cheese and half a punnet of berries
- 1 Laughing cow cheese on a wholewheat crackers
- Mini fruit smoothie, made with half a banana, 240 ml (8 fl oz) of milk, ice, cinnamon and a dollop of yogurt.

*Note: after the age of two years, kids can switch to low fat or no fat dairy products.

Is It Hunger or Is It a Craving?

You might be thinking that your child is going through a growth spurt because they are endlessly saying they're hungry, even after a substantial meal. If you can determine whether your child is genuinely hungry or is just having a craving, then it will be easier for you to recognize if they really do need more food, or if there is another reason why they're asking for it.

The difference between hunger and a craving is:

Hunger: a physiological response to the drop in blood sugar levels. Kids will eat almost anything you offer them if they are genuinely hungry. It can be harmful to ignore a hunger signal.

Craving: a psychological response to food based on boredom, emotions or its availability. A craving is usually for a particular food, and nothing else will suffice. There is no harm in ignoring a craving; in fact, it's probably very good to do so.

Use the following steps to determine whether your child is actually hungry or just having a craving:

- When your child asks for more food after they've just had an adequate meal or snack, ask them to go and occupy themselves for 20 minutes and then return.
- More often than not, they'll forget. However, if

they return still wanting food, offer them a healthy option such as a piece of fruit or yogurt.

- If they take the healthy option, then they are genuinely hungry.
- If they refuse the healthy option and want only a particular type of food, say "no" (there is no harm in this), and ask them to wait until the next meal or snack time.

The Five Food Groups

Every day, kids need a variety of foods from the five major food groups for optimum growth and development. Remember, the recommendations provided are purely for children, as their nutritional requirements are very different to adults because they are growing at such a rapid rate. These are general recommendations, so they may not apply to kids who have other health issues. If this is the case, we recommend you seek specific advice from a dietitian.

1. Grains: includes breads, cereal, rice, pasta and noodles

Grains are our fuel, particularly for our carb-hungry brains. They help kids have the energy to run around, concentrate at school, as well as grow taller.

Kids up to the age of 11 years need four to five servings a day, while those aged 11 to 18 years need four to seven servings of grains per day, depending on how active they are. One serving of grains is:

- 1 slice of bread
- ½ a wrap or flat bread
- 125 ml (4 fl oz) of rice, pasta, noodles, oats, quinoa, barley, buckwheat
- 150 ml (5 fl oz) (¼ pint) of flaked cereal
- 60 ml (2 fl oz) of muesli
- 3 crispbreads
- 1 crumpet or small English muffin.

2. Dairy: includes milk, yogurt and cheese

Dairy is the greatest and richest source of calcium and is in high demand for growing skeletons and for teeth.

Kids need 2½ to 3½ servings of dairy foods per day. One serving of diary is:

- 125 ml (4 fl oz) of milk or other dairy alternative or calcium-fortified milk
- 1 small tub of yogurt
- 2 small slices (40 g (1.4 oz)) of hard cheese

3. Vegetables

Vegetables contain the roughage from fiber for healthy bowel movements, plus precious vitamins and minerals to keep us healthy.

Kids need four to five servings of vegetables every day. One serving of vegetables is:

- 250 ml (8 fl oz) of salad

- 125 ml (4 fl oz) of cooked vegetables, corn kernels, cooked beans, lentils or legumes
- ½ medium potato
- 1 medium tomato

4. Fruit

Fruit provides all-important roughage, which is necessary for healthy bowel movements, plus vitamins and minerals that stop us from getting sick. They are also a source of natural sugar that work as fuel or energy for the body. Whole fruit is always better for us than fruit juice or added fructose (fruit sugar), as it contains fiber.

Kids need two servings of fruit each day. One serving is:

- 1 apple, orange, banana
- 2 smaller fruit like a kiwi fruit or plum or other stone fruit
- 110 g (4 oz) diced fruit (no added sugar or syrup)
- 30 g (1 oz) dried fruit
- 125 ml (4 fl oz) fruit juice (no sugar added)

5. Protein

Protein forms the building blocks for our body as it is necessary for the growth and repair of our muscles and organs; to create hormones; to support our immune system, and to carry oxygen around our body. When we eat foods that contain protein, our small intestine breaks down the food into individual pieces called amino acids. These amino acids can then be reformed and reused again in the body, depending on where the body needs them. There are many amino acids, but nine of them we are unable to make within our body so we must source them from the foods we eat. Foods that contain complete proteins have all of these essential amino acids and can be found in all animal products, like meat, fish, chicken, eggs, as well as dairy and soy.

Children need 1½ to 2½ servings of protein foods every day. One serving is:

- 100 g (3.5 oz) meat, chicken (uncooked weight)
- 120 g (4.2 oz) fish (of uncooked weight)
- 2 eggs
- 150 g (5 oz) cooked legumes or lentils
- 170 g (6 oz) tofu
- 30 g (1 oz) nuts or seeds or their paste (no added sugar or salt)

6. "Extra" or "Sometimes" Foods

"Extra" or "sometimes" foods are the sixth unofficial food group and are called this because they should be considered *extra* to our normal healthy diet of the five main food groups. This is because they contain little to NO nutritional value; in other words, they do nothing good for our body.

Some of these foods have a benign effect on

kids, as in, they aren't terribly nutritious but they are also not terribly harming. For example, good quality potato chips that are cooked in a healthy oil, a scoop of vanilla ice cream, or a couple of squares of dark chocolate are okay. Obviously too much of these foods will make it hard to maintain a healthy weight, but a little on occasion is just fine.

On the other hand, there are also some unhealthy extra foods, that are packed full of artificial colors, flavors, fillers, white refined sugars and flour. These foods should be severely limited, and even eliminated for kids with behavioral issues, allergies or intolerances. They are not only energy-dense and make maintaining a healthy weight very difficult, but they may also be quite harmful to your kids.

The over-consumption of this group of foods is often the cause of kids being overweight, obesity and ill health among children today. If these extra foods take the place of healthy, the result can include nutrient deficiencies, energy crashes, hyperactivity, immune system suppression (causing persistent colds and flu), slow recovery and wound healing, and in the long term it may even increase the risk of type 2 diabetes, cancers and heart disease – even at their young age.

Reading Food Labels

The first thing to understand when it comes to reading food labels is that the order the ingredients are listed is significant. This is because the order in which the ingredients appear on the label indicates how much of it is contained in that particular food. For example, if "whole milk" appears first in the list, then whole milk is the largest ingredient in that product. The second largest ingredient will then be the item that appears second in the list, and so on.

Learning to understand a food label is incredibly empowering because it allows you to determine immediately whether a particular packaged food is a healthy choice or a "sometimes" food. The benefit to teaching the kids to read labels is that they can help make decisions as to whether or not to buy the food. By involving them in the decision process, it may also lessen any potential conflicts that may arise when at the supermarket.

Checking food labels of packaged products is only necessary for non-staple foods. This is because staple foods are typically foods found in their most natural state, which are part of the traditional five food groups. For example, you would not need to check the food label of fresh bread, pasta, rice, meat, fruit or vegetables *unless* they had been processed in some way. If the food has been processed, it will generally have a nutrition panel and ingredients list on it (see nutritional panel image on page 70).

For those "extra" or "sometimes" foods that typically come in packaging, here is a helpful three-step rule to understanding food labels. Remember, although the packaged food may be promoted as being "healthy", it really is up to you to use the following three-step rule to decide whether the added ingredients (such as sodium and artificial flavors and colors) are something you're comfortable with your kids consuming.

NUTRITION INFORMATION
Servings per package: 3
Serving size: 150g

	Per serve	Per 100g
Energy	608kj	405kj
Protein	4.2g	2.8g
Fat, total	7.4g	4.9g
Saturated	4.5g	3.0g
Carbohydrates, total	18.6g	12.4g
Sugars	18.6g	12.4g
Sodium	90mg	60mg

Whole milk, concentrated skim milk, sugar, banana (8%), strawberry (8%), grape (4%), peach (2%), pineapple (2%), gelatine, culture, thickener (1442)

The three golden rules to reading food labels:

Step 1.

Look for "Fat, total" and view the far column which states the "Quantity per 100 g". This figure should read less than 5 g per 100 g. If not, this item should immediately be considered a "sometimes" food and you should move to Step 2.

Step 2.

Look for "Sugars" (not "Carbohydrates") and read the far column, again titled "Quantity per 100 g." If the figure is less than 5 g per 100 g, it is a packaged food that you can consider okay for your kids. If the sugars are greater than 5 g per 100 g, then go to Step 3.

Step 3.

If sugars are more than 5 g per 100 g, then you need to find out where the sugars are coming from. And this is because all sugars are not created equally! There are healthy sources of sugars that are acceptable for kids to eat, and there are refined, added sources of sugar which should be considered a "sometimes" food.

Food labels often use other names for *unhealthy* sugars. These include:

- sucrose
- maltose
- glucose
- fructose
- corn syrup
- brown sugar
- maple syrup
- honey
- high fructose corn syrup

Food labels may also use other names for *healthy* sugars, which include:

- fruit puree
- fruit concentrate
- milk
- milk solids
- yogurt

As we mentioned earlier, the ingredients list appears in order, with the biggest ingredient mentioned first, and the smallest ingredient appearing last. Start at the beginning and go through the ingredients until you come across a sugar. In the food label shown on page 70, it's listed as "sugar", so it's a refined, added source of sugar, deeming this product a "sometimes" food.

Be aware that healthy sugars can be found in fruit and dairy. So if, for example, the banana or strawberry ingredient is listed on the label before the sugar (or any of the commonly used terms above), then it means the majority of the sweetener in the food is from a natural source of sugar and could, therefore, be considered a food to add to a healthy diet.

It's OK To Say "No"

NIC SAYS

When it comes to our children's relationship with and behaviors around food, one of the biggest issues can be a parent's inability to say "no".

Without a doubt, there are times when we are busy and feel exhausted, and prefer to avoid a fight or a tantrum, so we give in to our kids. We totally get it. This is why the 80/20 rule is great; because there is a time and a place for "sometimes food" or a little extra food – you don't always have to say "no" to everything.

Of course, ultimately it's up to you to make those decisions for your kids. But keep in mind that the less often they have the treat, the more likely they will appreciate it even more. Saying "no" can help them learn why they need to eat nutritious foods, what is an appropriate size for a treat food, and how often it is OK for them to have it. If you think about this as being just like all the other battles you might have, such as going to bed at a certain time, having a shower, looking both ways before crossing the road or brushing their teeth, you can see that in the bigger picture it's just another decision for your kids' safety; it is in the best interest for their health. So instead of thinking that saying "no" is being mean, think of it as tough love that will teach them right from wrong, and help ensure that they are as healthy as can be – both now and in the future.

Creating An Ideal Day Of Eating

So let's put all this together.

There are many variations of this day and it's up to you to get a little creative so the kids (and you) don't get bored. On the opposite page is a template to help you create an ideal day of eating for the kids and keep a check on whether they are eating the right amount of each of the essential food groups.

The example chart opposite shows the following totals:

• Grains = 7 serves

• Dairy = 2½ serves

• Veggies = 5 serves

• Fruit = 2 serves

• Protein = 1½ serves

Food Allergies and Intolerances

Around 1 in 20 kids suffer from food allergies. Typically, they are caused by an immune response to a substance in particular foods. Most food allergies for kids are not severe and they usually grow out of them; however, some can be quite severe causing hives, eczema, swelling, wheezing and vomiting. Some allergies may even be life threatening, (e.g. anaphylaxis) and must be taken very seriously. This is the reason for banning particular foods from being brought into school or kindergartens, as it is a way to eliminate potential exposure of those sensitive

children, to that allergen. Common trigger foods for kids are eggs, cow's milk, peanuts, tree nuts, seafood, sesame, soy, fish and wheat.

In contrast, food intolerances are usually reactions to a sugar component in a food, such as lactose, milk sugar or other components of food such as gluten. Intolerances do NOT involve the immune system, but can cause headaches, upset tummies, bloating and problems going to the toilet. Unlike allergies, intolerances are not life threatening and therefore, will not be banned from schools. However, in most cases, eliminating these problem foods from a child's diet will be sufficient to manage their symptoms and sometimes it may also improve their behavior and reduce fussy eating.

The recipe and snack ideas we've included in the following section includes alternative foods that can be used if your kids suffer from allergies.

EXAMPLE IDEAL EATING CHART

Meal Time	What to Eat	Food Groups
Breakfast	2 slices of wholegrain toast 1 mini tin of baked beans Glass of milk	2 serves of grains 1 serve of veggies 1 serve of dairy
Lunchbox (including recess + lunch)	1 container of chopped veggie sticks + cherry tomatoes 1 wholegrain wrap with chicken + avocado 1 small tub of yoghurt 1 piece of fruit	2 serves of veggies 2 serves of grains ½ serve of protein 1 serve of dairy 1 serve of fruit
Afternoon Tea	4 Vitaweet crackers 1 slice of cheese	1 serve of grain ½ serve of dairy
Dinner	1 cup of basmati rice Small steak 1 cup of cooked veggies	2 serves of grains 1 serve of protein 2 serves of veggies
Dessert	Small bowl of chopped fruit	1 serve of fruit

CHAPTER
TEN

Everyday Recipes And Snacks They'll Love

Feeding time can be such a nightmare especially in today's world with allergies and fussy eaters. There is nothing worse than getting to THAT time of the day when a meal needs to be thought of or a lunch needs to be packed. Having been through the trials, successes and failures of feeding a family at the end of a stressful day, we have been able to come up with some absolute winning recipes that the kids and the parents will LOVE.

These recipes not only taste great, they are all nutritionally balanced and make feeding time, simple and more importantly quick to prepare. Busy parents, spend much of their time stressing about what to cook and how to make sure the family are eating well and healthily. In our recipes section you will find a recipe for all times of the day and in between.

No more thinking, no more stressing, just quick simple cooking and yummy eating.

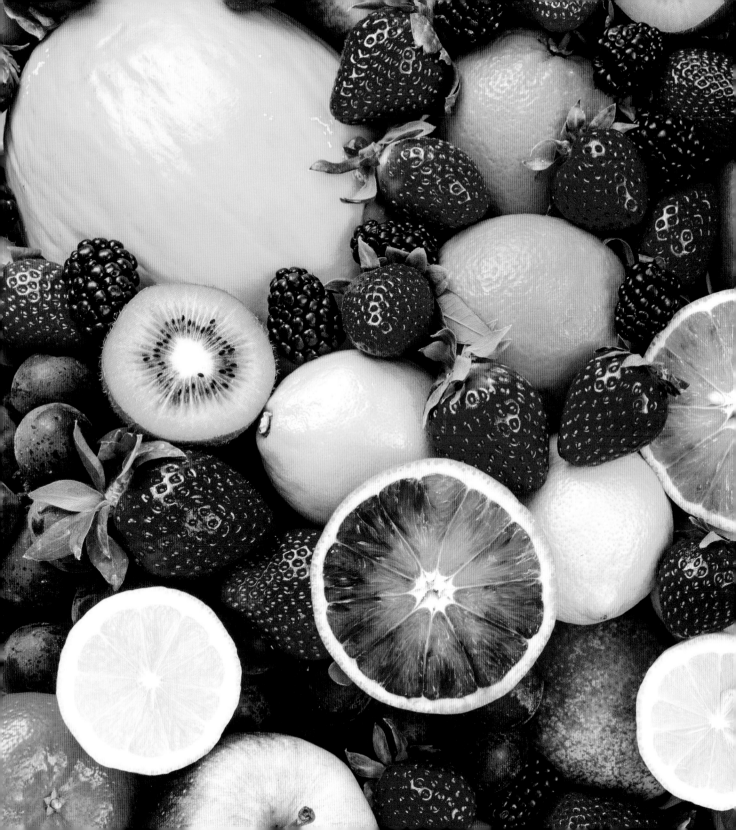

BREAKFAST

Scrambled Eggs and Ham Wrap

Serves: 2

YOU WILL NEED:

- 2 eggs
- Dash of milk (cow's, rice, oat, almond, goat or sheep milk)
- 80 to 100 g (2.8 to 3.5 oz) lean ham off the bone
- 2 thin wholemeal wrap bread or a gluten free wrap

METHOD:

1. In a bowl, beat together the eggs and milk until mixed well. Place the bowl in the microwave for 30 seconds. Take it out and mix it up with a fork, then place back in the microwave for another 30 seconds or until it is the consistency you like. Use a fork again to scramble in the bowl.

2. Divide out the ham and egg mixture, place on the bread, then roll 'em up! Slice into pinwheels for a fun and easy-to-eat shape.

Allergy notes:

- Egg allergy: as an alternative to the eggs you could use cottage cheese, lactose free or normal.
- Cow's milk allergy: use rice milk instead of cow's milk.
- Gluten or wheat allergy/ intolerance: use gluten free wrap.

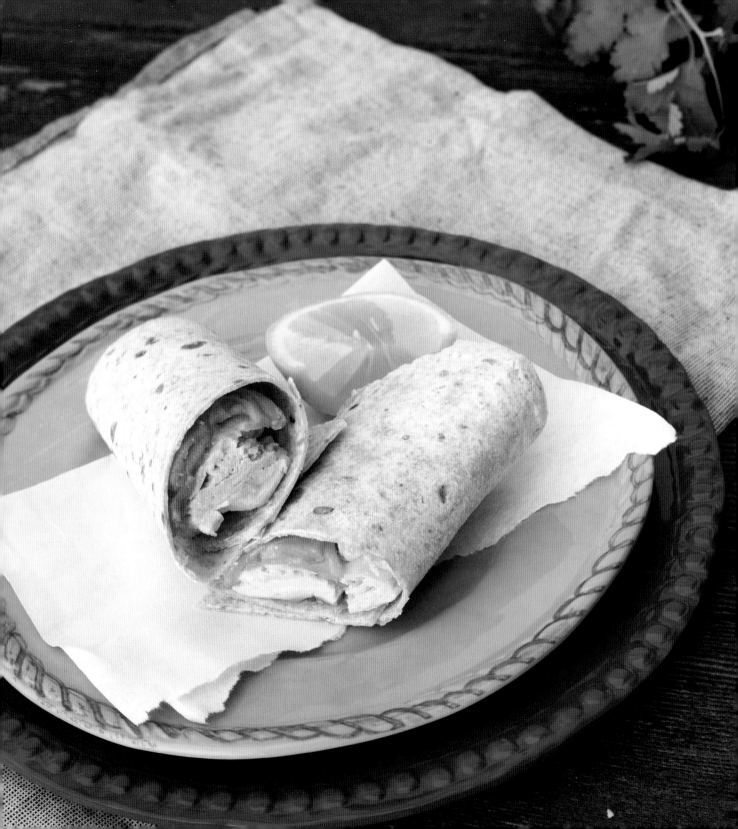

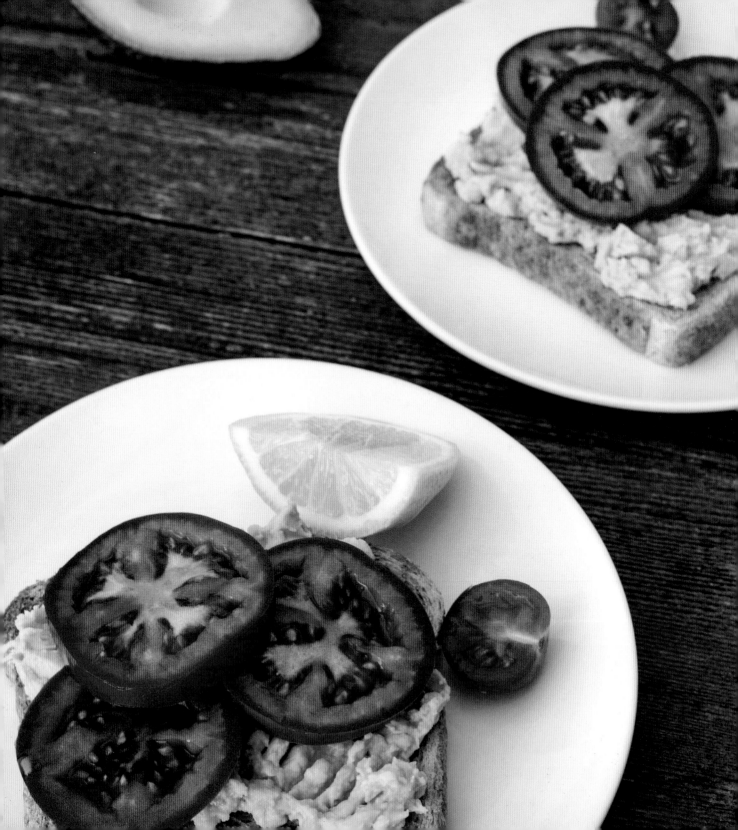

Smashed Avocado and Tomato on Toast

Serves: 2

YOU WILL NEED:

- 2 pieces of bread (wholegrain, wholemeal or gluten free)
- ½ avocado
- 1 tomato, sliced
- Squeeze of lemon

METHOD:

1. This is simple and quick, so there's no excuse to not start your day off right. Toast bread in a toaster (or if you prefer it fresh then leave it untoasted), and spread a half of the avocado on each slice of toast.

2. Top with some slices of fresh tomato.

3. Add a little squeeze of lemon juice, and it's ready to eat!

Allergy notes:

- Gluten allergy: use gluten free bread.
- Wheat allergy or intolerance: use 100 per cent rye, spelt, buckwheat, corn or kamut bread.

 5

Fat is the most essential nutrient for small kids. A little fat in the diet is as important as the vitamins.

A, D, E and K are fat-soluble vitamins, which means they can't be absorbed without having a little fat available.

Wholemeal Banana Mini Hot Cakes

Serves 4

YOU WILL NEED:

- 2 large bananas
- 375 ml (12 fl oz) wholemeal self-rising (self-raising) flour
- 375 ml (12 fl oz) full fat milk
- 2 eggs, lightly whisked
- 1 tablespoon honey or maple syrup
- Olive oil cooking spray
- ½ punnet of strawberries
- A reduced fat yogurt of your choice, to serve

METHOD:

1. Mash one banana in a bowl.

2. Put flour in a bowl and make a well in the center.

3. Combine milk, eggs, honey and mashed banana in a jug. Pour into the well and whisk until it is all combined. Stand for 10 minutes.

4. Heat a large, non-stick pan to medium heat and spray with a little oil. Spoon 60 ml (2 fl oz) of the hot cake mix into the pan. Cook for 2 to 3 minutes or until bubbles appear on the surface and then turn. Cook for 1 to 2 minutes on the other side. Transfer to a plate. Cover to keep warm.

5. Repeat with remaining batter to make 12 hot cakes.

6. Slice the second banana and the strawberries. To serve, place the hot cakes on plates and top with the sliced banana and strawberries and a couple of dollops of yogurt.

Allergy notes:

- Gluten allergy: use gluten free flour.
- Wheat allergy or intolerance: use gluten free flour, oat flour or 100 per cent rye or buckwheat flour.
- Dairy allergy: use rice milk instead of cow's milk and coconut yogurt instead of cow's yogurt.

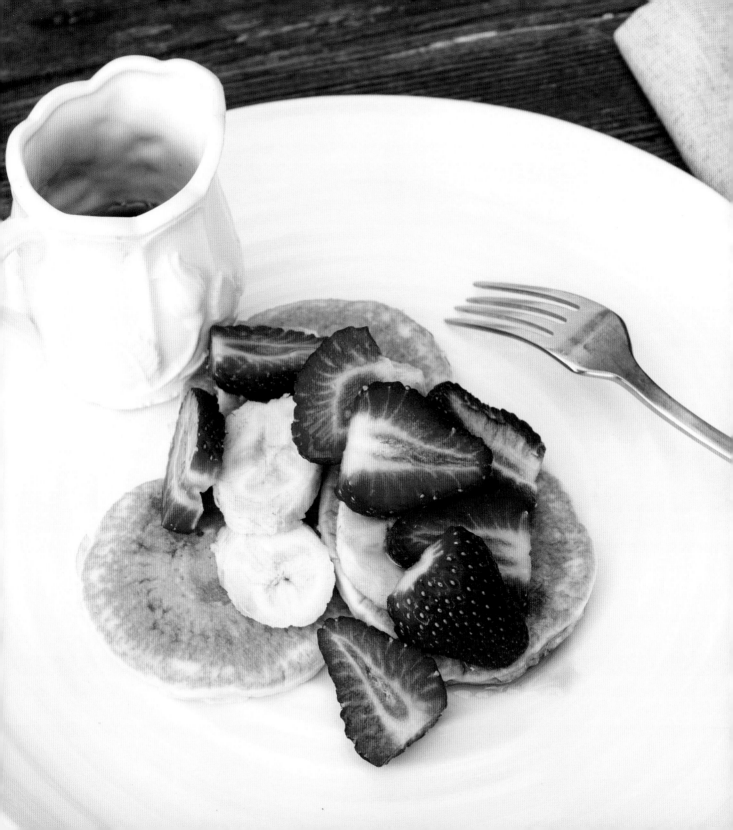

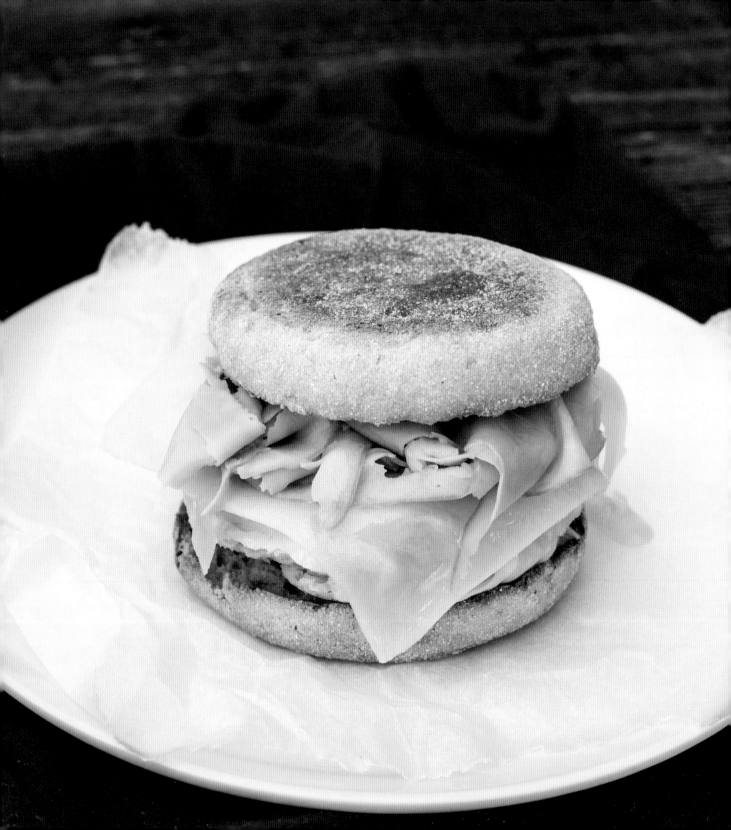

Ham and Egg English Muffins

Serves: 4

YOU WILL NEED:

- Olive oil spray
- 120 g / 4.2 oz shaved leg ham off the bone
- 4 eggs
- 4 wholegrain English muffins, halved and toasted
- 4 slices reduced-fat tasty cheese

METHOD:

1. Spray a frying pan with oil. Pan-fry ham, turning for a couple of minutes until light golden. Transfer to a plate and cover to keep warm.

2. Spray the pan with oil again and cook eggs for four minutes or until cooked to your liking.

3. Place four muffin halves on a baking tray lined with foil. Place one egg on each muffin and top each with ham and one slice of cheese. Grill for 1 minute or until the cheese has melted. Top with the remaining muffin halves.

Allergy notes:

- Gluten or wheat allergy or intolerance: use gluten free English muffins.
- Dairy allergy: omit the cheese or replace with lactose free.
- Egg allergy: as an alternative to the eggs you could use cottage cheese, lactose free or normal.

Oaty Banana Smoothie

Serves: 4

YOU WILL NEED:

- 125 ml (4 fl oz) traditional rolled oats
- 2 ripe bananas, frozen
- 500 ml (16 fl oz) reduced-fat milk
- 250 ml (8 fl oz) reduced-fat plain Greek-style yogurt
- 2 teaspoons honey
- 250 ml (8 fl oz) ice cubes

METHOD:

1. Blend all ingredients together until smooth. Pour between two large glasses and enjoy!

Allergy notes:

- Gluten allergy: omit the rolled oats and use quinoa flakes as an alternative.
- Dairy allergy: use rice milk instead of cow's milk and coconut yogurt instead of Greek yogurt.

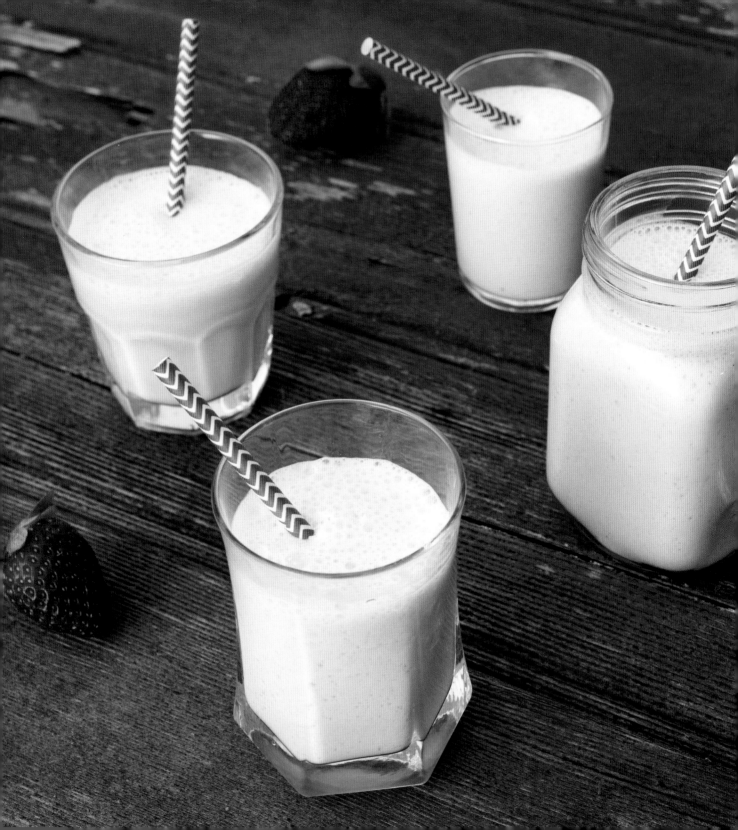

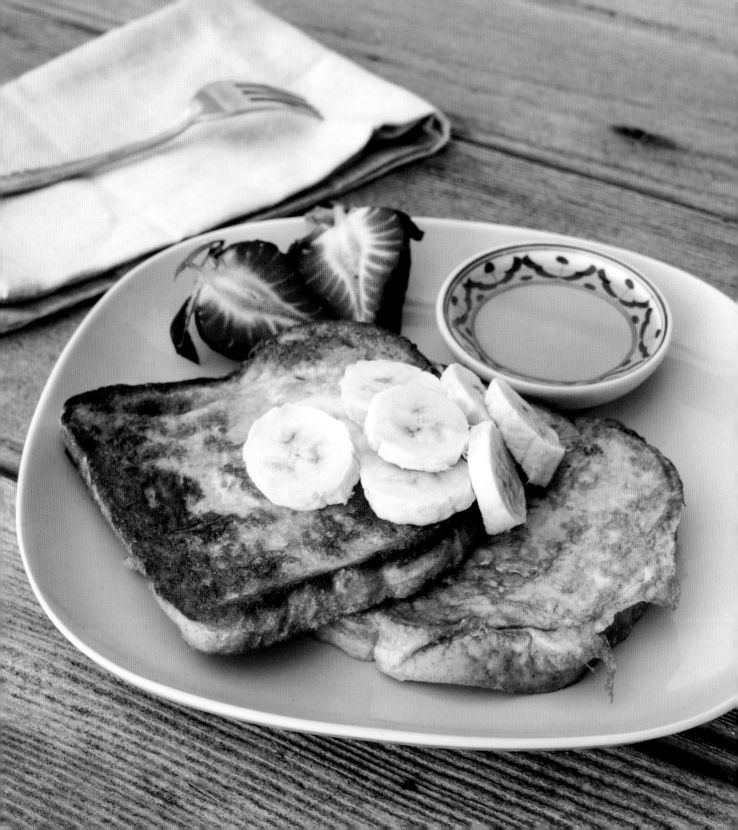

Coconut French Toast

Serves: 4

YOU WILL NEED:

- 4 eggs
- 270 ml (9 fl oz) can light coconut milk
- ½ teaspoon ground cinnamon
- 1 tablespoon honey
- 25 g (1 oz) butter
- 8 slices fresh wholemeal or wholegrain bread
- 2 large bananas, sliced
- 250 ml (8 fl oz) plain Greek-style yogurt
- 2 tablespoons honey for serving

METHOD:

1. Preheat oven to 150°C (300°F) and line a baking tray with baking paper.

2. Whisk eggs, coconut milk, cinnamon and honey together in a shallow dish.

3. Melt 1 teaspoon of the butter in a large frying pan over medium heat. Dip two slices of bread in the egg mixture until soaked through, draining any excess egg mixture and place into the pan. Cook bread for two to three minutes each side or until golden.

4. Transfer to the oven tray and keep in the oven to stay warm. Repeat with the remaining slices of bread, egg mixture and butter.

5. Divide toast between two plates and serve with sliced banana, a few dollops of yogurt and honey.

Allergy notes:

- Egg allergy: this recipe is not appropriate for people who have an egg allergy.
- Gluten allergy: use gluten free bread.
- Wheat allergy or intolerance: use gluten free bread or 100 per cent rye or oat bread.
- Dairy allergy: dairy free spread instead of butter and coconut yogurt instead of Greek-style yogurt.

LUNCH AND DINNER

Lamb Cutlets with Steamed Vegetables

Serves: 2

YOU WILL NEED:

- 1 tablespoon olive oil

- 4 lamb cutlets

- 1 zucchini (courgette) per person, thickly sliced

- 1 carrot, thickly sliced

- 1 bell pepper (capsicum), sliced

- 1 teaspoon butter (or dairy free spread)

- Squeeze of lemon

METHOD:

1. Heat a frying pan on a medium to high heat. Drizzle the olive oil to coat each lamb cutlet. Place the cutlets into the frying pan and cook on one side for around 3 to 5 minutes, until golden brown. Flip them over and cook for another couple of minutes on the other side until cooked through and browned on each side.

2. While the lamb is cooking, bring a steamer to the boil and add the zucchini and carrots (and any other vegetables you like) and steam until they are tender. This should take about 4 to 5 minutes.

3. Top the vegetables with a teaspoon of butter and a squeeze of lemon juice, give them a mix and distribute them between two plates along with the sliced bell pepper. Add the lamb cutlets to the plates and watch the kids tuck in!

Allergy notes:

- For cow's milk allergy: use dairy free spread

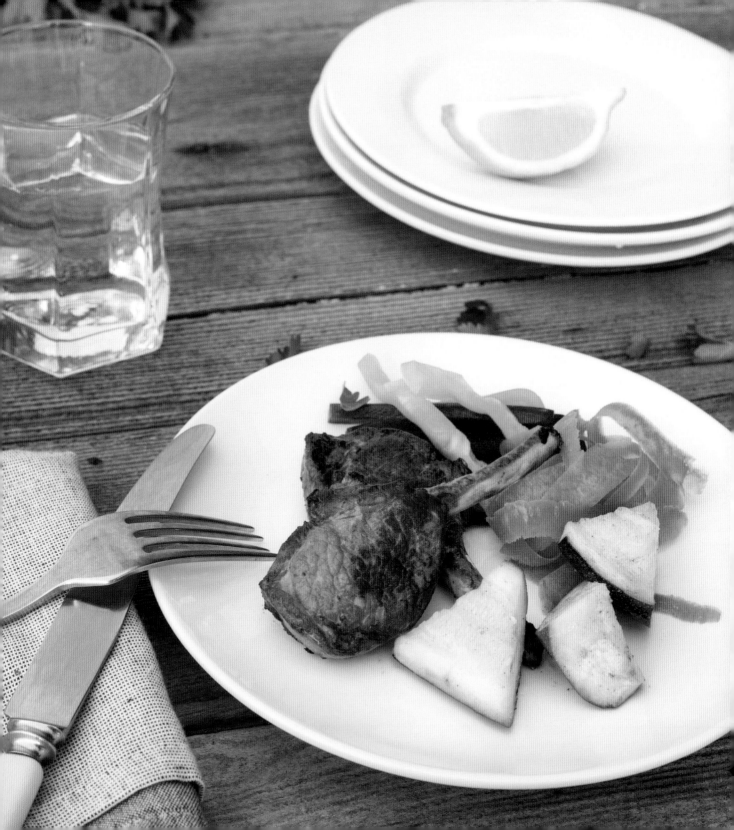

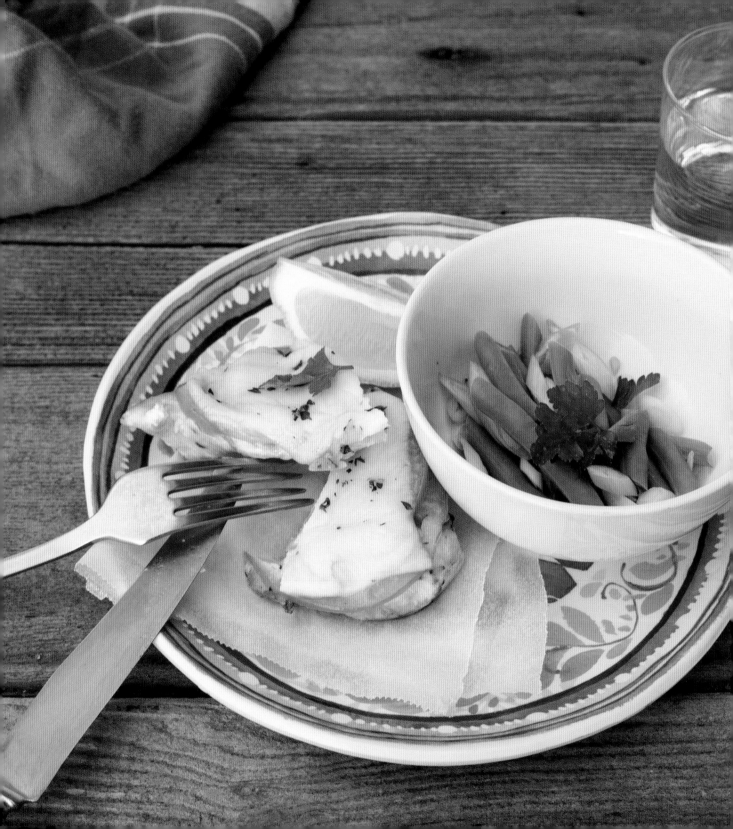

Healthy Chicken Parmagiana (they won't even know!)

Serves: 2

YOU WILL NEED

- 1 large chicken breast fillet
- Dried Italian herbs (optional)
- Olive oil
- ½ small avocado
- 1 large tomato, thinly sliced
- 2 slices of reduced fat cheese
- 20 green beans, with the ends removed
- 2 tablespoons of olive oil
- 1 teaspoon vinegar (white, balsamic or apple cider)

METHOD:

1. Slice the chicken breast in half to make it thinner or cover the chicken with a plastic bag or baking paper and using a meat mallet, bang out the chicken until its half the thickness. Sprinkle with a little Italian dried herbs.

2. Heat a frying pan on medium to high heat and add a drizzle of olive oil and the chicken, searing it on both sides until they start to brown.

3. Put the grill on high and place the chicken pieces onto a sheet of baking paper. Top with sliced avocado, tomato and a slice of cheese and place under the grill for a few minutes or until the cheese melts and begins to bubble.

4. Place the beans in a bowl with a dash of water, cover with cling wrap and microwave for 1 minute. Take the beans out, drain and allow to cool. Drizzle the beans with a little olive oil and vinegar or lemon juice.

5. To serve, on each plate place a chicken piece and half the beans. YUM!

Allergy notes:

- Cow's milk allergy: omit cheese or replace with lactose free.

Chilli Bean Nachos – A Vegan's Delight

Serves: 4

YOU WILL NEED:

- Olive oil
- 1 brown onion, diced
- 1 clove of garlic, minced
- Pinch of salt
- 1 large carrot, grated
- 1 zucchini (courgette), grated
- 1 stick of celery, finely diced
- 1 can of red kidney beans
- 1 can of black beans or white beans
- 1 x 400 ml (13.5 fl oz) tin of diced tomato
- 1 teaspoon dried mixed Italian herbs or dried oregano
- 2 teaspoons good quality stock powder
- 1 tablespoon tomato sauce (choose variety with no added sugar)
- 375 ml (12 fl oz) of cooked rice (preferably brown or basmati)
- 1 large avocado
- ½ lemon, juiced
- 1 small tomato

METHOD:

1. Heat a large pan on medium to high heat and add a drizzle of olive oil, then the onion and garlic and a pinch of salt. Stir for a couple of minutes until the onion begins to soften.

2. Add the carrot, zucchini and celery and continue to stir and cook for a further 5 minutes.

3. Add the tinned beans and tomato to the vegetables, dried herbs, stock and tomato sauce. Stir to combine. Bring the bean mix to the boil, then reduce to a simmer and partially cover with a lid. Allow the chilli beans to reduce down for around 20 minutes.

4. Whilst the beans are cooking, make the guacamole by mashing the avocado and lime juice in a bowl, then stir through the tomato.

5. To serve, divide the rice between two bowls, top with a couple of big spoonfuls of chilli beans and a big dollop of guacamole.

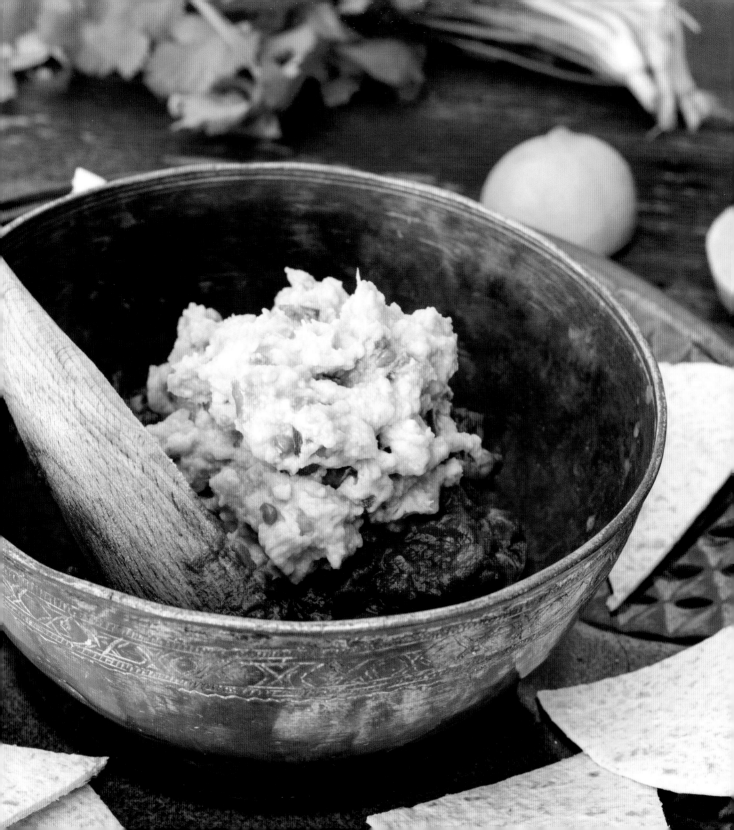

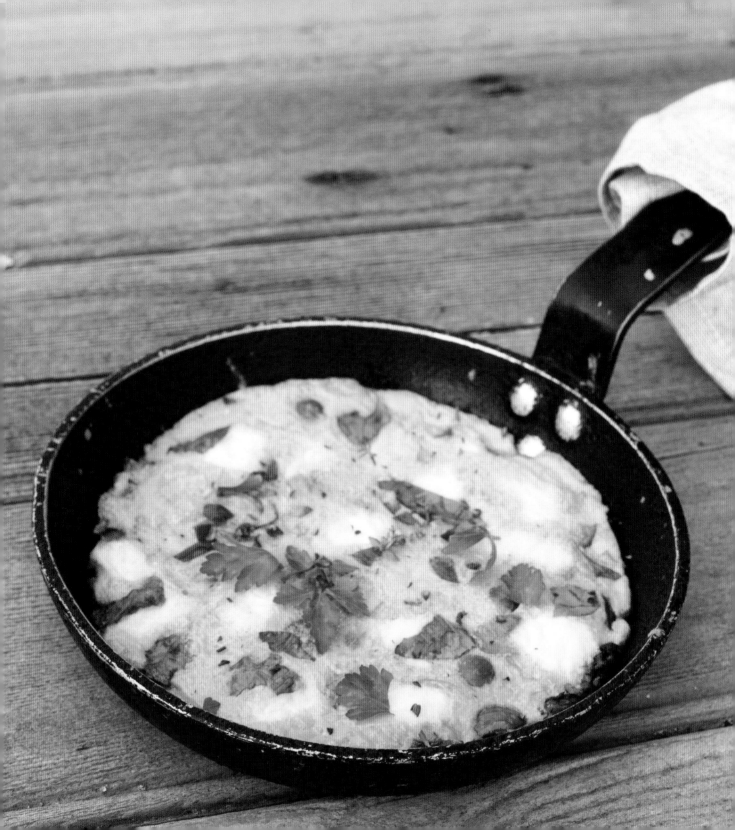

Mediterranean Frittata – Another Vegetarian's Delight

Serves: 4

YOU WILL NEED:

- 3 whole eggs (free range and preferably organic)
- A dash of milk (reduced fat, soy, rice or almond milk)
- Sprinkle of Parmesan cheese, to taste
- Olive oil
- ¼ Spanish onion, diced

- 6 to 8 pitted black olives, chopped
- Handful of baby spinach, chopped into shredded pieces
- 3 small cubes of feta cheese
- 2 slices of toast (wholegrain, wholemeal, gluten free)

METHOD:

1. In a mixing bowl beat the eggs with the milk, and Parmesan cheese.

2. Turn on your oven grill to a high heat. Heat a small frying pan on medium to high heat, drizzle a teaspoon of olive oil and add the onion until soft.

3. Slowly pour the egg mixture into the frying pan and reduce the heat a little.

4. Sprinkle over the olives and spinach and crumble the feta evenly across the egg mixture. Let the bottom of the frittata cook slowly, for around 5 minutes. Use an egg flip to check and see if it the bottom has become brown.

5. Once it has browned, place the whole frying pan under the grill to cook the top.

6. Cut the frittata in half or quarters and enjoy on top of a slice of the toast of your choice. This frittata is also great for breakfast or dinner or cold for lunch!

Allergy notes:

- Egg allergy: this recipe is not appropriate for an egg allergy.
- Cow's milk allergy: omit the Parmesan and feta cheese, use a dash of rice milk instead of cow's milk.
- Gluten allergy/ intolerance: use gluten free bread.
- Wheat allergy/ intolerance: use 100 per cent rye or gluten free bread.

Homemade Sang Choy Bow

Serves: 2

YOU WILL NEED:

- 250 g (9 oz) chicken mince (you can also use pork or turkey mince)
- 1 tablespoon olive oil
- 1 clove of garlic
- 1 teaspoon of chopped ginger
- 4 scallions (spring onions)
- 125 ml (4 fl oz) of chopped mushrooms

- 1 small tin of corn (or chopped baby corn)
- 5 green beans, chopped
- 125 ml (4 fl oz) of frozen or fresh peas
- 1 tablespoon ketchup manis (sweet soy sauce), tamari or soy sauce
- Splash of sesame oil
- 4 iceberg lettuce cups

METHOD:

1. Make sure all ingredients are chopped up into small pieces and ready to go, before you start heating the pan.

2. Place the oil in a frying pan (or wok if you have one) and heat for a minute, before adding the garlic, ginger and scallions (and chili is optional). Cook for around one minute, then add the chicken mince and cook while constantly stirring and mixing.

3. Once the mince has cooked through, add in all the chopped vegetables and all the sauces, stirring for a few minutes until the sauces are mixed through.

4. Place a few big spoonfuls inside the iceberg lettuce cups, fold the ends over, roll in the sides and enjoy!

Note: This recipe makes around four or so portions, so is ideal for two people. Just double the amounts to feed more people!

Allergy notes:

- Soy allergy: omit the ketchup manis, you can use a pinch of salt if you like.
- Sesame allergy: omit the sesame oil.

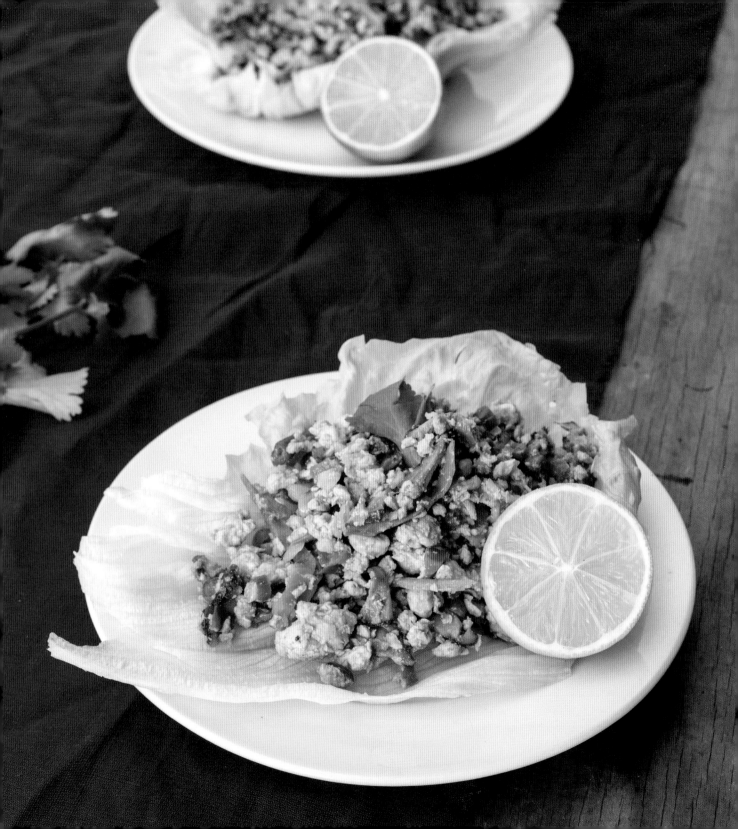

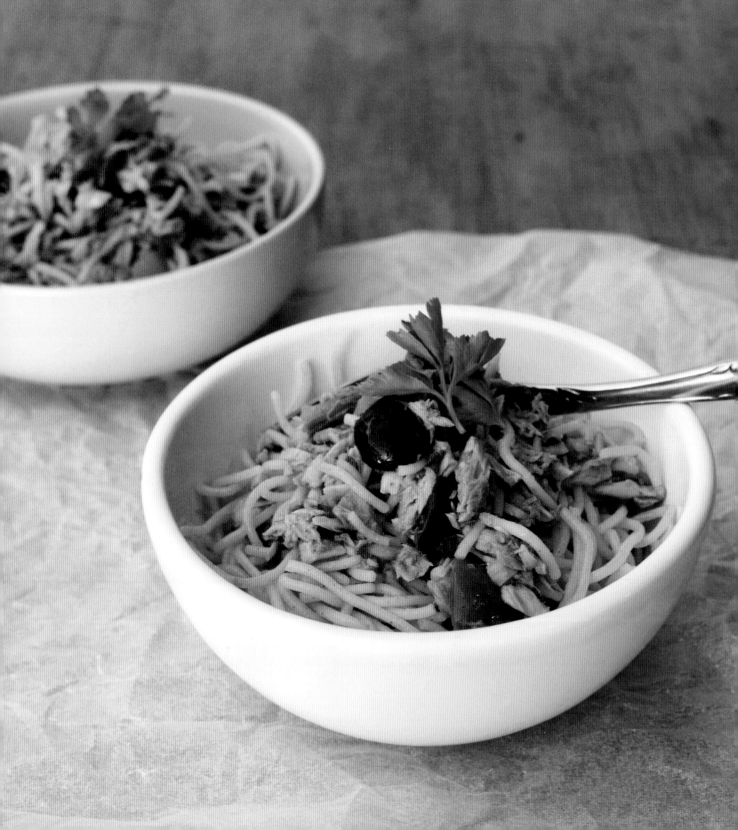

Peasant Pasta

Serves: 2

YOU WILL NEED:

- Angel hair pasta* (gluten free options are available).
- Small tin of tuna in olive oil
- 1 clove garlic, chopped
- 10 cherry tomatoes, each cut in half

- Handful of basil, chopped
- 4 black olives, chopped
- ½ teaspoon of sugar
- Sprinkle of Parmesan cheese
- Salt and pepper to taste

METHOD:

1. Using the olive oil from the tuna tin, coat the bottom of the frying pan and heat. Add in the garlic and tuna, cook for a few minutes, then add in the tomatoes, basil and olives.

2. Add the salt, pepper and sugar and bring to the boil for 1 minute, turn down and simmer for 10 minutes.

3. While simmering, boil the water to cook the pasta. Once boiling, add in the pasta and cook until al dente.

4. Drain the pasta and then add it to the frying pan with the sauce. Stir through until all pasta is well coated.

5. Serve with fresh lettuce leaves or on its own with a sprinkle of Parmesan cheese.

Note: A per person serve is best worked out by forming a circle with your thumb and index finger. The ring should be about 1 inch. The amount of uncooked pasta that fits through this circle is typically sufficient for one person. This recipe can also be made with brown rice replacing the pasta.

Allergy notes:

- Gluten allergy: use gluten free, quinoa, rice, corn or buckwheat pasta.
- Wheat allergy or intolerance: use gluten free, quinoa, rice, corn, buckwheat or rye pasta.
- Fish allergy: omit the tuna, you can use chicken, beef, lamb or pork instead or just keep it vegetarian.
- Dairy allergy: omit the Parmesan.

Honey, Soy Chicken with Rice Noodles and Beans

Serves: 2

YOU WILL NEED:

- 1 packet of vermicelli rice noodles
- 1 tablespoon of olive oil
- 1 garlic clove, chopped finely
- 1 small piece of ginger, chopped finely
- 1 chicken breast fillet or 2 thigh fillets per person, chopped into bite-sized pieces
- 2 tablespoons of soy sauce
- 1 tablespoon of honey
- 125 ml (4 fl oz) of chicken stock
- A big handful of green beans, chopped into bite-sized pieces

METHOD:

1. In a bowl, place vermicelli noodles in cold water and leave for 10 minutes.

2. In a hot pan (or wok) heat oil with garlic and ginger for a minute and then add in chicken pieces. Panfry chicken pieces until all are golden brown.

3. Add soy sauce, honey and chicken stock, then let simmer for 5 minutes.

4. Drain the noodles leaving 2 tablespoons of the liquid, which you can add to the pan with the beans. Toss the noodles and beans through until nicely coated (around 5 minutes), then serve.

Note: This is an easy-to-prepare recipe, which tastes even better if you can marinate the chicken pieces overnight.

Allergy notes:

- Soy allergy: omit the soy sauce.

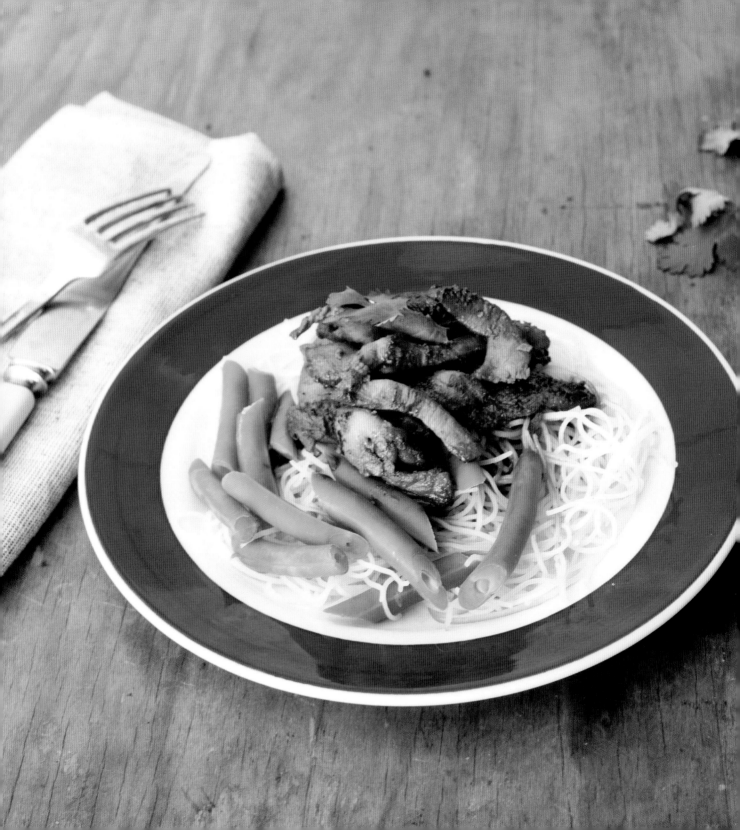

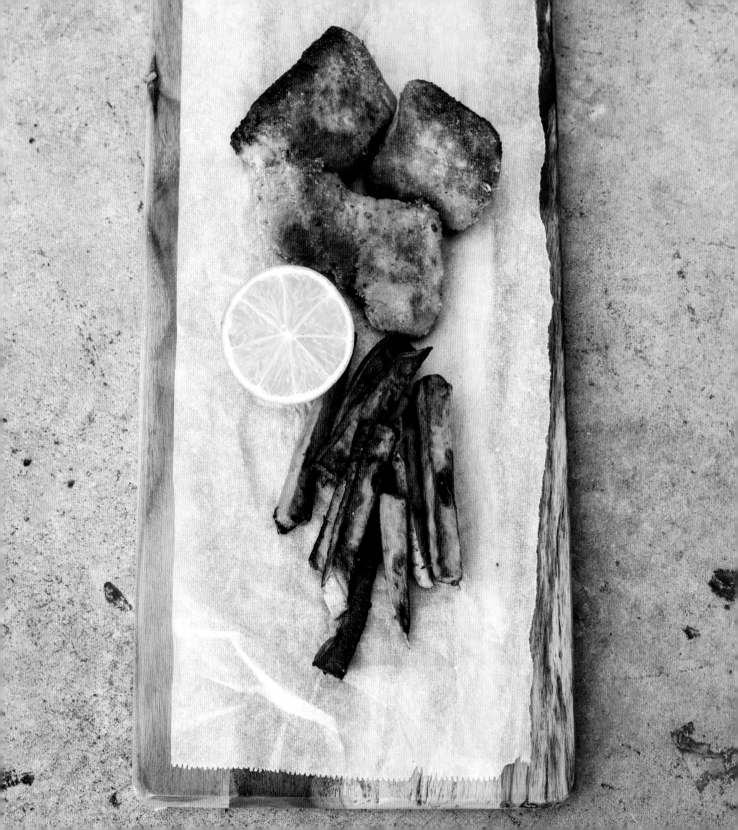

Homemade Fish Fingers and Yogurt Seafood Sauce, with Sweet Potato Chips

Serves: 2

YOU WILL NEED:

- 1 piece of your favorite fish per person (ling fillets and salmon fillets work well)
- 1 big piece of sweet potato
- 125 ml (4 fl oz) of any type of flour
- 2 eggs
- Breadcrumbs
- Handful of Parmesan cheese

- Olive oil for frying

Seafood Sauce

- 50 g (2 oz) of plain yogurt
- Tomato sauce
- 1 tablespoon Worcestershire sauce
- Juice of lemon

METHOD:

1. Preheat the oven to 180°C (350°F).

2. Slice the sweet potato into thin chip size pieces and par boil for 5 minutes. Drain, cool and set aside.

3. For the seafood sauce, place a dollop of plain low fat yogurt in a small bowl, add a squeeze of tomato sauce, the Worcestershire sauce and a squeeze of lemon. Mix and place into the fridge.

4. Place the flour, beaten eggs and breadcrumbs in three separate bowls, mixing a handful of Parmesan cheese into the breadcrumbs. Cut your fish into finger-style pieces and coat each piece in the flour, eggs and breadcrumbs.

5. When you are about to start cooking the fish, place your sweet potato chips in a baking dish with a little olive oil, salt and pepper and place them in the preheated oven. Cook the sweet potato chips until golden brown.

6. Coat the bottom of the frying pan with olive oil over a medium heat. Cook the fish at a medium rate until each side is a nice dark golden brown and then remove from heat.

7. Take the chips out of the oven and serve alongside the fish and salad, with a lemon wedge and seafood sauce.

Allergy notes:

- Fish allergy: use chicken tenderloins instead of fish.
- Gluten allergy: Gluten free, rice or corn flour. Gluten free bread crumbs. Gluten free Worcestershire sauce.
- Dairy allergy: omit the Parmesan and use plain coconut yogurt instead of Greek-style yogurt.
- Egg allergy: omit the egg.

Baked Chicken Nuggets

Serves: 4

YOU WILL NEED:

- 125 ml (4 fl oz) plain flour
- 2 eggs, lightly whisked
- 250 ml (8 fl oz) dried wholegrain breadcrumbs
- 500 g (17.5 oz) chicken tenderloins
- Olive oil spray

METHOD:

1. Preheat oven to 200°C (400°F) and line an oven tray with baking paper.

2. Place the flour, egg and breadcrumbs in separate shallow bowls. Season the flour with salt and finely ground white pepper.

3. Place the chicken into the flour and gently toss to coat. Dip a chicken piece into the egg then press into the breadcrumbs to coat.

4. Place on the lined tray and repeat with remaining chicken pieces. Lightly spray the crumbed chicken with oil spray and bake in the preheated oven, turning occasionally, for 10 to 12 minutes or until golden brown and cooked through.

Allergy notes:

- Gluten allergy: use gluten free, rice or corn flour. Use gluten free or rice breadcrumbs.
- Egg allergy: omit the egg, you can use a mixture of flaxseed meal mixed into water instead.

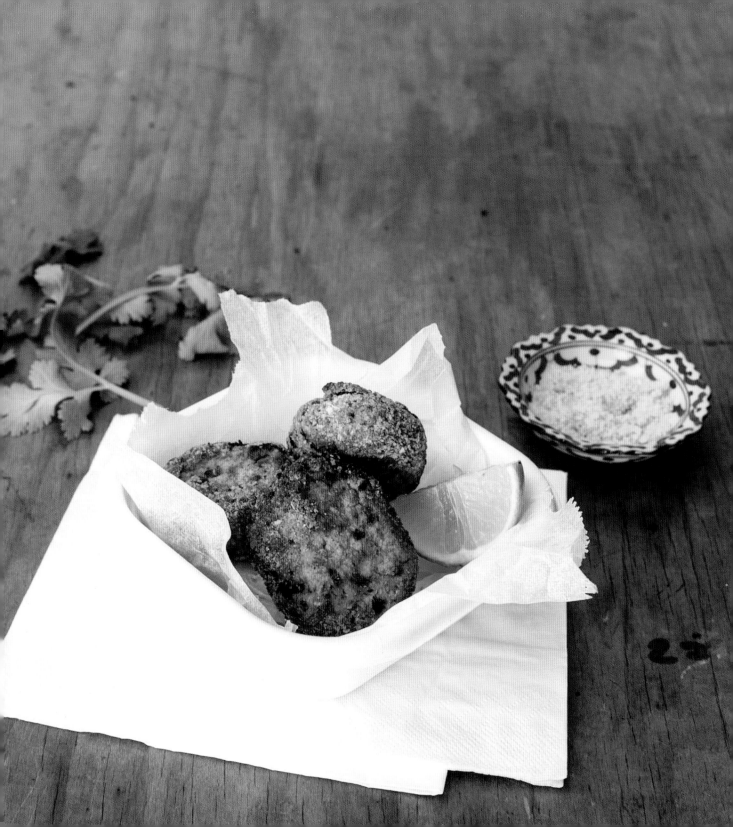

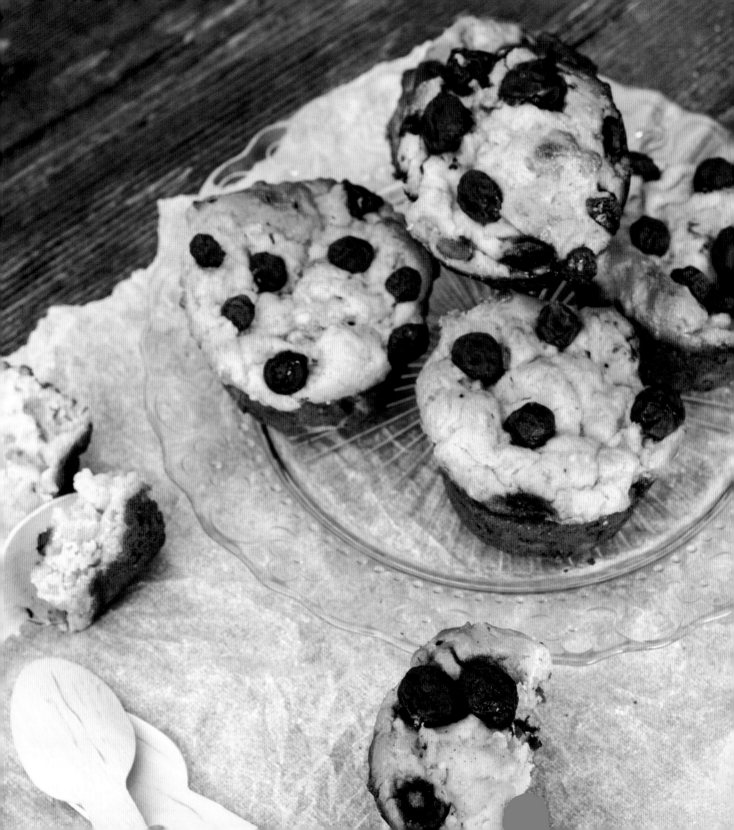

NOT-SO-NAUGHTY SNACKS

Yogurt Muffins with Banana and Berries
Makes: 12

YOU WILL NEED:

- 625 ml (20 fl oz) wholemeal plain flour, almond meal or gluten free flour
- 1 teaspoon baking powder (gluten free)
- 1 teaspoon ground cinnamon
- 60 ml (2 fl oz) maple syrup or honey
- 250 ml (8 fl oz) banana, mashed
- 1 teaspoon vanilla extract
- 1 egg, lightly beaten
- 425 ml (14 fl oz) reduced-fat yogurt
- 60 ml (2 fl oz) extra-light olive oil
- 125 ml (4 fl oz) frozen blueberries

METHOD:

1. Preheat oven to 170°C (325°F) and line a 12-hole muffin pan with paper cases.
2. In a large bowl, combine flour, baking powder, cinnamon and maple syrup and make a well.
3. Add banana, vanilla extract, egg, yogurt and oil, stir until combined.
4. Spoon into paper cases and top with blueberries.
5. Bake for 20 to 25 minutes until golden on top and when a skewer is entered, it comes out clean.
6. Stand in pans for two minutes then transfer to a wire rack to cool.

Allergy notes:

- Gluten or wheat allergy: use gluten free flour or almond meal.
- Nut allergy: use gluten free or wholemeal flour instead of almond meal.
- Egg allergy: use egg replacer (such as Orgran 'No Egg').
- Dairy allergy: use coconut yogurt instead or cow's yogurt.

Cheese and Tomato Muffins

Makes: 12

YOU WILL NEED:

- 625 ml (20 fl oz) wholemeal self-rising (self-raising) flour
- 250 ml (8 fl oz) grated reduced-fat tasty cheese
- 125 ml (4 fl oz) marinated sun-dried tomatoes, drained, chopped
- ½ teaspoon salt
- 300 ml (10 fl oz) (½ pint) reduced fat milk
- 1 egg, lightly beaten
- 90 g (3.2 oz) butter or dairy-free spread, melted

METHOD:

1. Preheat oven to 180°C (350°F) and lightly grease a 12-hole non-stick muffin pan.

2. Sift flour into a large bowl and add cheese, tomatoes and salt. Stir to combine making a well in the center.

3. In a seperate bowl combine the milk, egg and butter then pour the mixture into the well in the flour mixture. Using a large spoon, stir until just combined, but be careful not to over-mix.

4. Spoon mixture into muffin holes until three-quarters full. Bake for 20 minutes or until a skewer inserted into the middle comes out clean. Allow to cool in the pan for 1 minute, then place on a wire rack for further cooling.

Allergy notes:

- Gluten or wheat allergy: use gluten free flour.
- Dairy allergy: this recipe is not appropriate for a dairy allergy.
- Egg allergy: use 1 tablespoon flaxseed meal mixed with 2 tablespoons water instead of egg.

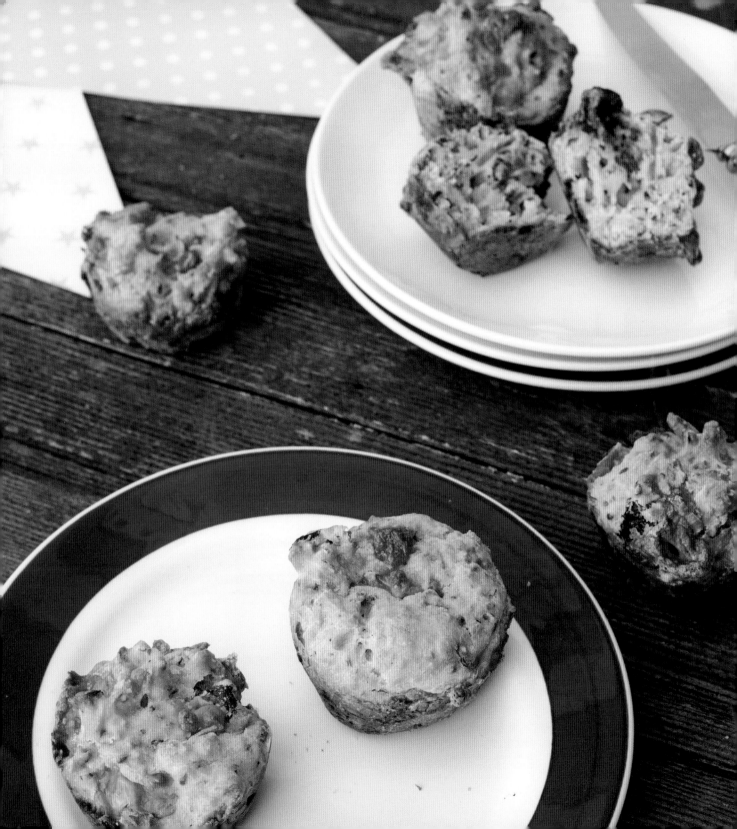

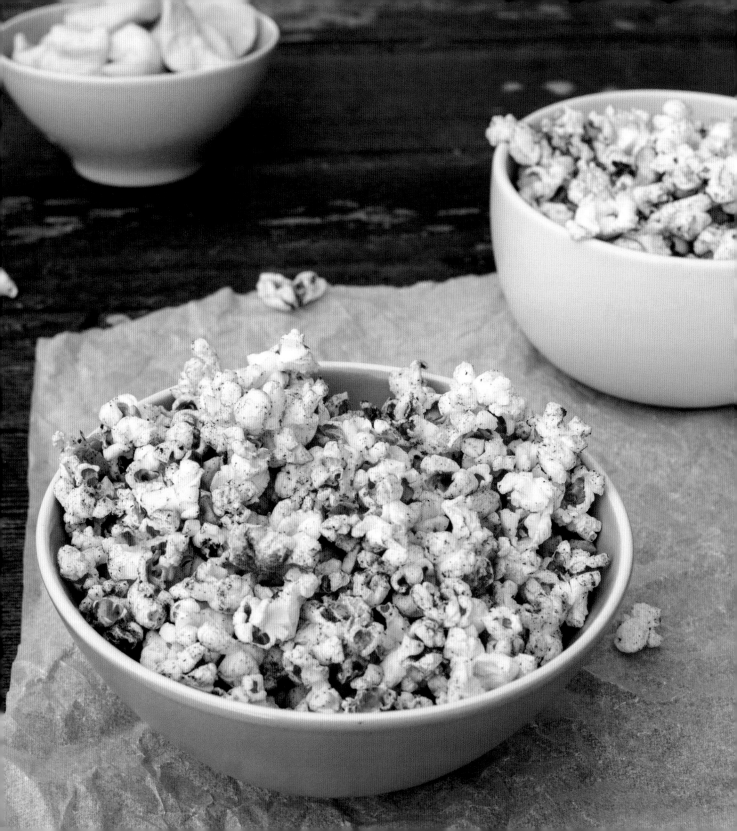

Apple and Cinnamon Popcorn

Serves: 4

YOU WILL NEED:

- 100 g (3.5 oz) packet of popcorn kernels
- 1 heaped tablespoon butter, melted
- 1 heaped teaspoon ground cinnamon
- 125 ml (4 fl oz) dried apple, chopped

METHOD:

1. Cook the popcorn kernels according to their packet instructions.

2. In a large bowl, add melted butter, cinnamon and the dried apple.

3. Toss popcorn into the apple and cinnamon mix until it's coated in the mix and enjoy!

Allergy notes:

- Dairy allergy: use dairy free spread instead of butter.

Seedy Apricot Bliss Balls

Makes: 12

YOU WILL NEED:

- 500 g (17.5 oz) dried apricots
- 60 ml (2 fl oz) hot water
- 60 ml (2 fl oz) shredded coconut
- 4 tablespoons peanut butter or other nut paste
- 60 ml (2 fl oz) honey
- 1 tablespoon cocoa powder
- 60 ml (2 fl oz) sesame seeds
- 150 g 5 oz) pepitas or sunflower seeds
- 60 ml (2 fl oz) chia seeds
- 80 g (3 oz) rolled oats

METHOD:

1. Line a large tray with non-stick baking paper.

2. Place half the apricots in a heatproof bowl and cover with the hot water and soak for 20 minutes.

3. Drain the apricots and place in a food processor with coconut, peanut butter, honey and cocoa powder and pulse until it forms a thick paste.

4. Finely chop the remaining apricots and place in a bowl with sesame seeds, pepitas, chia seeds, oats and apricot paste, mix well to combine. With damp hands, roll heaped tablespoons of mixture into balls and place on the prepared tray.

5. Refrigerate for at least one hour or until firm.

Allergy notes:

- Tree nut or peanut allergy: this recipe is not appropriate for nut allergies.
- Gluten allergy: use rice or quinoa flakes instead of rolled oats.

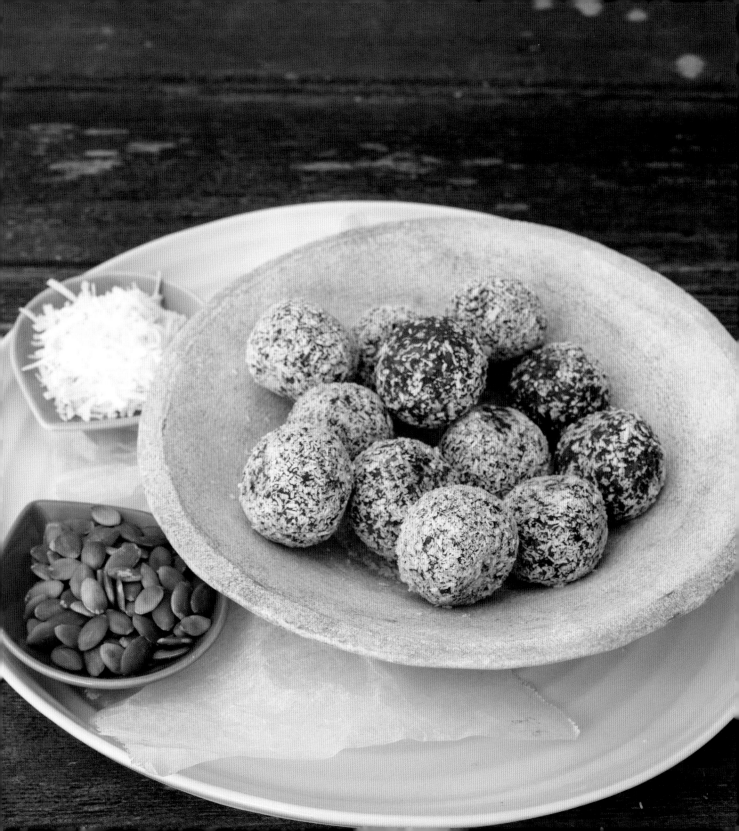

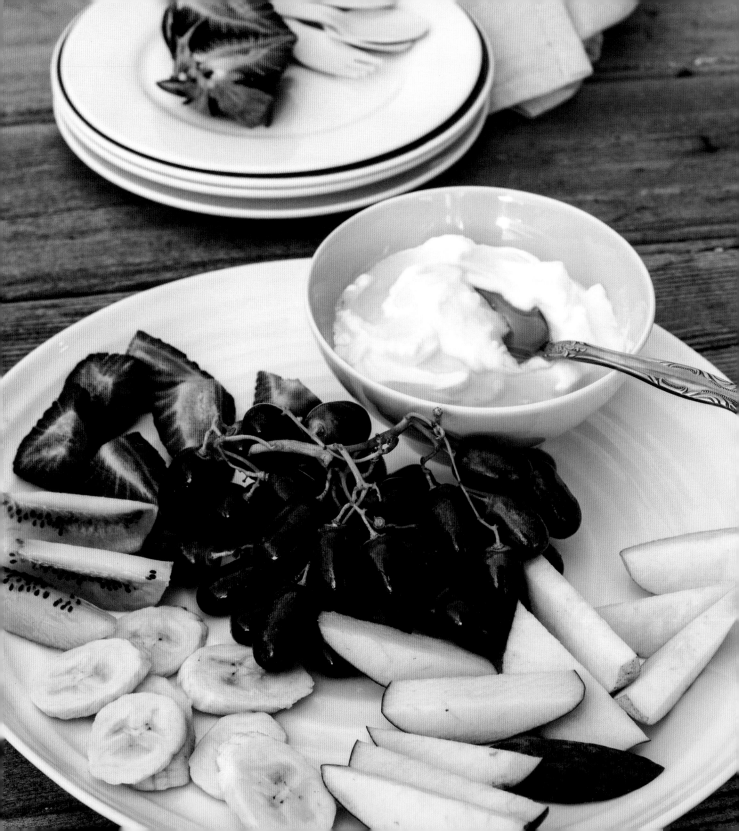

Yogurt Fruit Dip

Serves: 6

YOU WILL NEED:

- 200 g (7 oz) low-fat banana honey yogurt
- 1 red delicious apple, cored, cut into thin wedges
- 1 banana, peeled, sliced
- 1 small bunch (100 g / 3.5 oz) red and green grapes
- 1 small pear, skin removed and sliced
- 6 strawberries, topped and cut in half

METHOD:

1. Place yogurt into a small bowl. Place the bowl on a plate and display fruit around the bowl.

2. Using a fork, dip fruit pieces in the yogurt.

Allergy notes:

- Dairy allergy: use coconut yogurt instead or cow's yogurt.

Broccoli Trees

Serves: 4

YOU WILL NEED:

- 50 g (2 oz) flaked almonds
- 300 g (1 oz) broccoli, cut into small florets
- 80 g (3 oz) light cream cheese

METHOD:

1. Preheat oven to 180°C (350°F).

2. Place almonds on a baking tray and bake for 4 minutes or until golden and toasted. Set aside to cool.

3. Bring a large saucepan of water to the boil over high heat. Cook broccoli for 2 to 3 minutes or until bright green and tender. Drain, then refresh in a bowl of chilled water. Drain again and place on a large plate, and place almonds in a shallow dish and cream cheese in a small bowl.

4. Serve broccoli topped with cream cheese and press into the almonds.

Allergy notes:

- Dairy allergy: use cashew cheese instead of cream cheese.
- Tree nut allergy: if using cream cheese, then omit the flaked almonds.

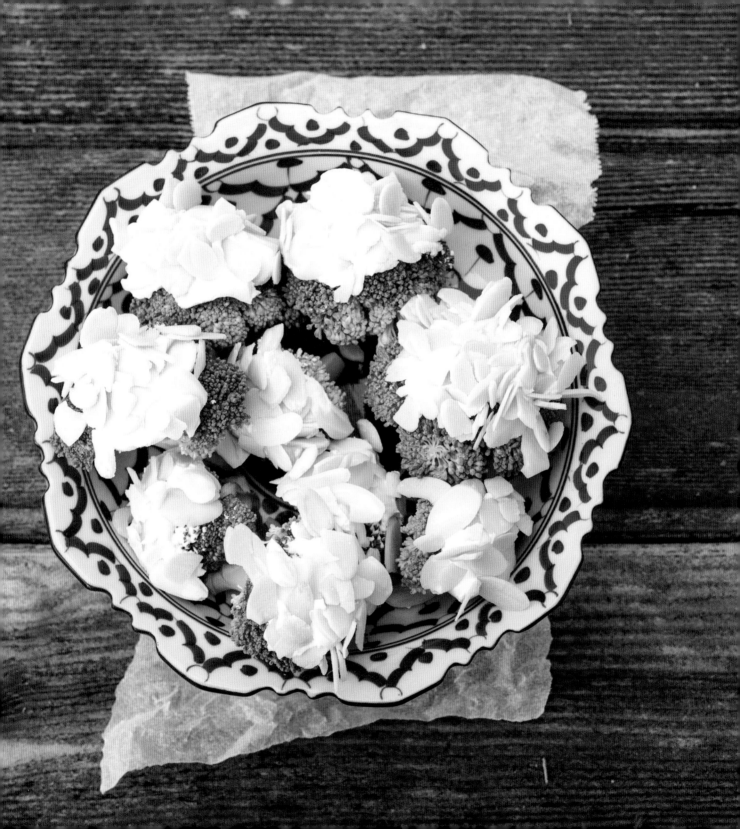

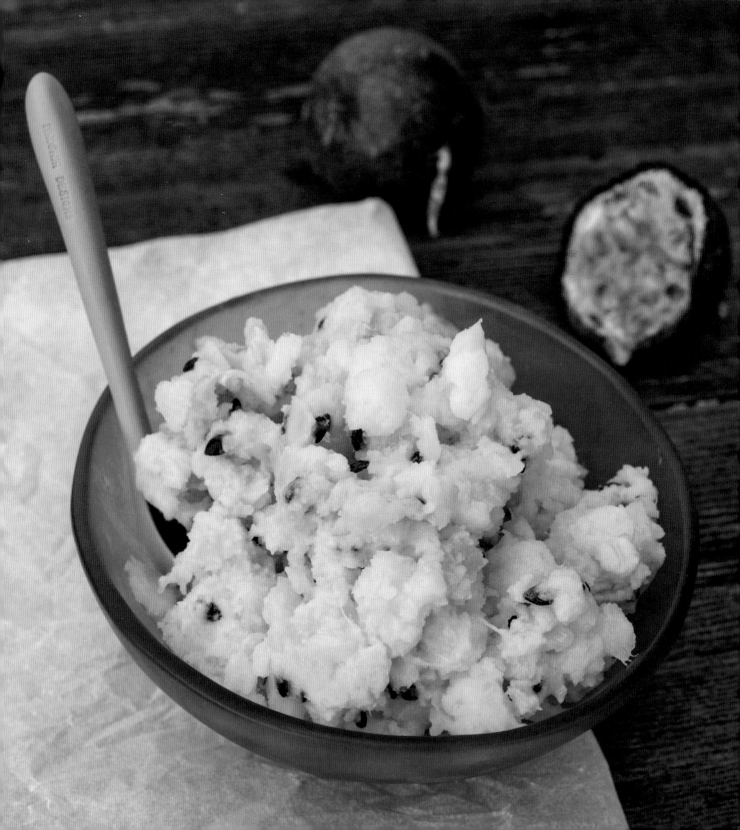

Frozen Pineapple Orange Crush

Serves: 4

YOU WILL NEED:

- 1 pineapple, peeled, cored and roughly chopped
- 2 oranges, peeled and chopped
- 80 ml (2.5 fl oz) fresh, frozen or tinned passionfruit pulp

METHOD:

1. Place pineapple, oranges and the passionfruit pulp in the bowl of a food processor and process until smooth.

2. Pour into a large shallow airtight plastic container. Cover and place in the freezer.

3. Mash with a fork every 3 hours, for 10 hours or until set.

4. To serve, use a fork and scrape the surface into coarse crystals. Divide among serving bowls and serve immediately.

Baked Tortilla Chips And Avocado Dip

Serves: 4

YOU WILL NEED:

- 4 small wholemeal pita bread pockets or corn tortillas
- Olive oil cooking spray
- 1 teaspoon paprika
- 1 large avocado, chopped
- 1 small tomato, deseeded, finely chopped
- 2 tablespoons lime juice
- Pinch of salt

METHOD:

1. Preheat oven to 200°C (400°F).

2. Spray one side of each pita bread with oil and sprinkle each with a quarter teaspoon of paprika, seasoning with salt and pepper.

3. Cut each bread into 8 triangles and place in a single layer on 2 large baking trays. Bake for 8 to 10 minutes, swapping trays after 4 minutes or until bread is crisp. Transfer to a wire rack to cool.

4. While the pita chips are baking, skin and remove the seed of the avocado and mash it in a small bowl. Stir in the tomato, lime juice and salt. Enjoy dipping the crunchy chips in the avocado dip.

Allergy notes:

- Gluten or wheat allergy: use 100 per cent corn tortillas instead of pita pockets.

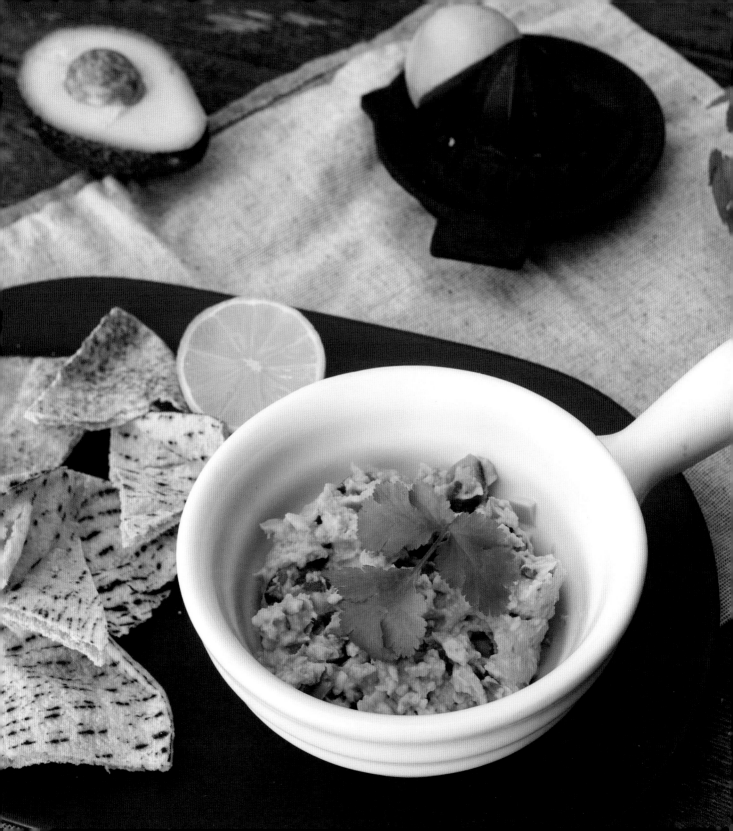

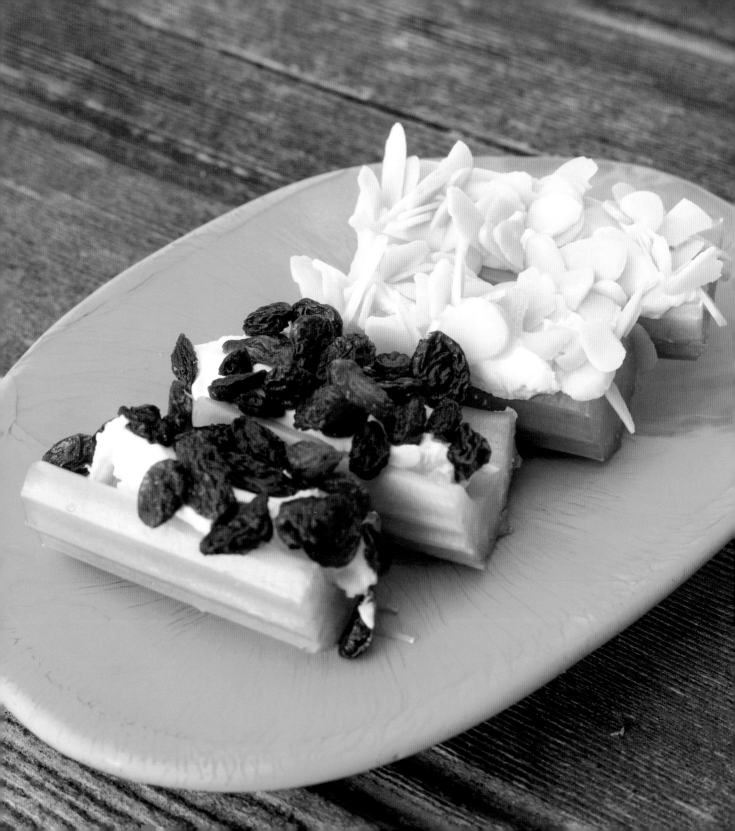

Celery Boats

Serves: 4

YOU WILL NEED:

- 6 long celery sticks
- 60 ml (2 fl oz) light Philadelphia creamed cheese
- 60 ml (2 fl oz) nut paste (natural peanut butter, almond paste, cashew spread)
- 4 tablespoons flaked almonds
- 4 tablespoons sultanas

METHOD:

1. Take the celery sticks and trim the ends, then cut each stalk into 3 pieces.

2. Fill each celery boat with either creamed cheese or nut spread, then dunk into the sultanas or flaked almonds and enjoy!

Allergy notes:

- Dairy allergy: omit the creamed cheese, you can use cashew cheese instead if you don't have a tree nut allergy .
- Peanut or tree nut allergy: omit the nut paste and omit the flaked almonds.

PART FOUR

Don't Stress Out!

CHAPTER
ELEVEN

Tips To Keep It Relaxed and Fun

"Life's Not Meant to Be A Chore"

Every day should be based around healthy eating and activities, as this will teach your kids what should be their "normal" way of living. Of course, the frequency and amount of "extra" foods consumed may vary when there are special occasions, weekends, vacations, staying at a friend's house, birthday parties, or the like. But, just like an adult, extra or "sometimes" foods should be reserved for these extraordinary occasions and events.

If these foods are limited in this way they are not seen as every day foods, your child will learn to associate these "sometimes" foods with special occasions and will appreciate them for what they are. If we're being really honest most kids have a sleepover or a birthday party every weekend, so keeping these treats to weekends is a great idea.

The next step is to discuss and agree on some boundaries around this, because it's easy to do a lot of damage during just one event, or over a busy weekend. So here are some golden rules:

Food should NEVER be used as a reward

By ensuring that kids do not use food as a reward for good behavior, they will avoid learning to use it to soothe themselves after a tough day or an emotional time. This is a terrible habit that contributes to many weight problems in adulthood. By teaching kids early, that there are non-food related ways to reward or self-soothe can go a long way to help save them a lifetime of weight-related issues. Non-food rewards could include:

- Sleepovers
- Magazines
- Extra pocket money
- Football cards
- Stationary
- Skipping rope
- Swimming accessories

It's important that our kids learn how to deal with disappointments. Here are some ideas to help you achieve this without them turning to food for comfort.

- Speak to kids with an even tone. If you're upset with them, wait until you have calmed down and go for a walk before reacting. Stop and ask yourself the question of "What do I want to achieve from this conversation?" Once you have your answer you will then find it easier to discuss the issue. One of the best tricks I learned when running big businesses was to count to 100. It's a simple technique that really works. I remember using it many times at the office, and now I often find myself stepping outside and counting to 100 when the children are pushing my boundaries. All it does is bring your energy levels back down by allowing your mind to focus on something else. This then provides you with some clarity. My mother was right when she said "you'll catch more flies with honey than with vinegar!"

- Sit down and explain that it's okay to have a bad day, as this is how we learn.

- To make sure it doesn't happen again, ask if there's anything you can help them with.

- Come up with a plan on how to deal with the problem or situation, if it occurs again.

- Include the behavior in your chart or diary for that week, as this will help with behavior change.

- Be a good role model by doing what you say you will do. Kids will mimic and pick up everything you do so the more you do with the kids in terms of activity and healthy eating, the less conflict there will be and the easier it will be for the kids to adapt your habits. By keeping it relaxed and fun you'll find things flow much more calmly and easily. By incorporating this into your everyday life, your behaviors will become second nature for both you and the kids.

- Each week, take turns so that a family member chooses an activity and their favorite meal. This way everyone feels included in the decisions that are being made.

- Get friends and family involved in your activities and meals. Kids are usually less fussy with their food and more active when other kids are around.

- Keep an "activity box" in the house that is full of games, props, dress ups, cards, exercise equipment like a skipping rope, so the kids can always be occupied. This means they're less likely to be asking about food and regardless of the weather or how busy you are, or how much space you have available at home, the kids will always have access to something to do.

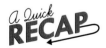

a Quick **RECAP**

When it comes to nutrition and eating:

- Everyone in the family needs to eat healthily.

- All meals and snacks should be eaten at the table: make mealtime a family conversational activity.

- Do not use food as a reward or punishment.

- Involve children in meal planning and grocery shopping; if children are involved in the decision-making, they are more likely to want to stick with a change in their routine.

- Keep healthy snacks on hand.

127

PART FIVE

Let's Join The Dots

CHAPTER
TWELVE

Bringing It All Together – Easily!

"Your Quick Start Guide"

- Start with the 80/20 Diary.
- Customize your own 80/20 Diary using our template on page 133 in the Annexures.
- Work together with your kids to develop their diary. Make it colorful and fun.
- Let them decide their rewards and points system. You can customize your own Rewards and Points System Charts using our templates on page 134 in the Annexures.
- Work together to design the chart and display it where it's visible everyday.

- Stay present. When you catch them doing something right, praise in public.
- Remember to reprimand in private.
- Keep the positive behavior loop going and it will, eventually, keep itself going.
- The responsibility to change habits is all yours. So stay on target for 21 days.
- Along the way remember to have fun, be playful and make them laugh as much as you can. Games make it all much easier, so turn up the fun factor whenever you can.

- Participate as much as possible as it strengthens your bond and shows them that you care. They'll realize that if it's good enough for you, then it's good enough for them.

- Build strength using their natural body movement and weight.

- Stretching doesn't take long but really can make a huge difference. A few minutes every day is all it takes.

- A stretch before bed helps relax their body and promotes a better quality sleep.

In terms of nutrition, make sure you educate yourself in the basics of kids' nutrition – remember, the more you know the healthier you and your kids will be. Here are our top 10 nutrition tips for healthier and happier kids:

1. Golden rule: don't use food as a reward. Use activities or other items as rewards.

2. Have breakfast before leaving the house, or take something that can be eaten on the way.

3. If it's not water or milk the kids are drinking, it's a treat (that's juice, soda, cordial, sports drinks).

4. The best snacks are made of a combination of carbohydrate and protein.

5. Make at least one really nutritious snack per day, and ensure this is consumed at their hungriest time of the day.

6. Make sure lunch and dinner meals are made up of at least a third vegetables or salad.

7. Dessert is not necessary. When you do have it, choose healthy options as well, such as fruit instead of ice cream.

8. For carbohydrate foods (rice, bread, pasta, noodles, crackers, cereals), the more brown and grainy in appearance, the better they will be for you.

9. Low fat dairy is fine from the age of two.

10. Make sure the kids' food portions are appropriate in size. They should not look like an adult-sized serving.

FINAL WORDS

At the start of this book, we asked you if you'd like to have a healthy and active family, who has the energy to do all the things they want to, and the enthusiasm to set and achieve goals throughout life? We posed the question of whether you'd like to understand how to help your kids (and the rest of the family – including yourself) flourish and thrive, to become healthy and successful for the rest of their life?

We acknowledged that many parents worry about their child being one of the larger kids at the park, or one of the biggest in the class. We hope that now you are at the end of this book you feel somewhat reassured that you are not alone and that even though parenting can feel extremely overwhelming at times, you are now armed with the knowledge and skills to reclaim your health and the health of your family with some simple, yet effective strategies.

Our final parting words of advice are to never underestimate the power of being a good role model. It's one thing to tell your kids *how* to live, but it's entirely different (and a lot more powerful) to do it yourself. Really believe in what you're doing, even if sometimes you may not like or enjoy it, and watch them copy and mimic you. You may not realize this, but you set the standard for your kids without uttering a single word. So practice what you preach and before long it will become the norm at home.

By using the 80/20 principle in all your thinking, we hope you'll realize that even though life isn't perfect and none of us are ever going to be able to deliver 100 per cent, 100 per cent of the time, you can regain your power and confidence, then the health and happiness of your family will be restored and maintained – for life!

REFERENCES AND FURTHER READING

For more information, review these references:

- Australian Bureau of Statistics. 2014
- Australian Institute of Health and Welfare. 2015
- Baechle, Thomas R. 2007.*Essentials Of Strength Training And Conditioning*.
- DeVries, Herbert A and Housh, Terry J. 2009. *Physiology Of Exercise*.
- Marieb, Elaine N. 1992. *Essentials Of Human Anatomy And Physiology (4th Edition)*.
- *Obesity: A National Epidemic And It's Impact On Australia*. 2014
- Weinberg, Robert S and Gould, Daniel. 1999. *Foundations Of Sports And Exercise Psychology*.
- http://synapse.org.au/get-the-facts/what-is-positive-behaviour-support-fact-sheet.aspx
- http://dictionary.reference.com/browse/positive+feedback
- http://kidshealth.org
- http://allergy.org
- http://www.who.int/growthref/en/
- http://www.who.int/growthref/bmifa_girls_z_5_19_labels.pdf?ua=1
- http://www.ncbi.nlm.nih.gov/pubmed/8483856

ANNEXURES

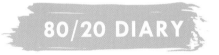

80/20 DIARY

Time	My Tasks	✔
		☐
		☐
		☐
		☐
		☐
		☐
		☐
		☐
		☐
		☐

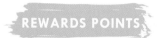

REWARDS POINTS

Task	Value	Mon		Tues		Wed		Thurs		Fri		W/end	
		C1	C2	C1	C2	C1	C2	C1	C2	C1	C2	C1	C2

REWARDS POINTS

Task	Value	Mon		Tues		Wed		Thurs		Fri		W/end	
		C1	C2	C1	C2	C1	C2	C1	C2	C1	C2	C1	C2

134

First published in 2016 by New Holland Publishers Pty Ltd
London • Sydney • Auckland

The Chandlery Unit 704 50 Westminster Bridge Road London SE1 7QY United Kingdom
1/66 Gibbes Street Chatswood NSW 2067 Australia
5/39 Woodside Ave Northcote, Auckland 0627 New Zealand

www.newhollandpublishers.com

A record of this book is held at the British Library and the National Library of Australia.

ISBN 9781742578064

Managing Director: Fiona Schultz
Publisher: Diane Ward
Project Editor: Holly Wilsher
Designer: Andrew Quinlan
Production Director: Olga Dementiev
Printer: Toppan Leefung Printing Limited

10 9 8 7 6 5 4 3 2 1

Keep up with New Holland Publishers on Facebook
www.facebook.com/NewHollandPublishers